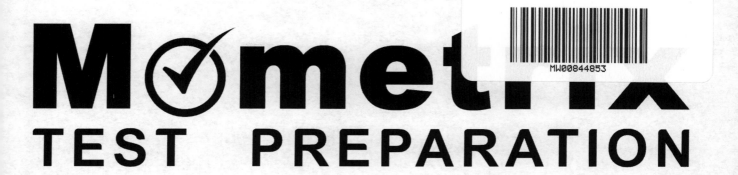

# Occupational
# Therapist
## Exam Secrets
## Study Guide

# DEAR FUTURE EXAM SUCCESS STORY

First of all, **THANK YOU** for purchasing Mometrix study materials!

Second, congratulations! You are one of the few determined test-takers who are committed to doing whatever it takes to excel on your exam. **You have come to the right place.** We developed these study materials with one goal in mind: to deliver you the information you need in a format that's concise and easy to use.

In addition to optimizing your guide for the content of the test, we've outlined our recommended steps for breaking down the preparation process into small, attainable goals so you can make sure you stay on track.

We've also analyzed the entire test-taking process, identifying the most common pitfalls and showing how you can overcome them and be ready for any curveball the test throws you.

Standardized testing is one of the biggest obstacles on your road to success, which only increases the importance of doing well in the high-pressure, high-stakes environment of test day. Your results on this test could have a significant impact on your future, and this guide provides the information and practical advice to help you achieve your full potential on test day.

**Your success is our success**

**We would love to hear from you!** If you would like to share the story of your exam success or if you have any questions or comments in regard to our products, please contact us at **800-673-8175** or **support@mometrix.com**.

Thanks again for your business and we wish you continued success!

Sincerely,
The Mometrix Test Preparation Team

---

**Need more help? Check out our flashcards at:**
**http://MometrixFlashcards.com/NBCOT**

---

# TABLE OF CONTENTS

# Introduction

**Thank you for purchasing this resource**! You have made the choice to prepare yourself for a test that could have a huge impact on your future, and this guide is designed to help you be fully ready for test day. Obviously, it's important to have a solid understanding of the test material, but you also need to be prepared for the unique environment and stressors of the test, so that you can perform to the best of your abilities.

For this purpose, the first section that appears in this guide is the **Secret Keys**. We've devoted countless hours to meticulously researching what works and what doesn't, and we've boiled down our findings to the five most impactful steps you can take to improve your performance on the test. We start at the beginning with study planning and move through the preparation process, all the way to the testing strategies that will help you get the most out of what you know when you're finally sitting in front of the test.

We recommend that you start preparing for your test as far in advance as possible. However, if you've bought this guide as a last-minute study resource and only have a few days before your test, we recommend that you skip over the first two Secret Keys since they address a long-term study plan.

If you struggle with **test anxiety**, we strongly encourage you to check out our recommendations for how you can overcome it. Test anxiety is a formidable foe, but it can be beaten, and we want to make sure you have the tools you need to defeat it.

# Secret Key #1 – Plan Big, Study Small

There's a lot riding on your performance. If you want to ace this test, you're going to need to keep your skills sharp and the material fresh in your mind. You need a plan that lets you review everything you need to know while still fitting in your schedule. We'll break this strategy down into three categories.

## Information Organization

Start with the information you already have: the official test outline. From this, you can make a complete list of all the concepts you need to cover before the test. Organize these concepts into groups that can be studied together, and create a list of any related vocabulary you need to learn so you can brush up on any difficult terms. You'll want to keep this vocabulary list handy once you actually start studying since you may need to add to it along the way.

## Time Management

Once you have your set of study concepts, decide how to spread them out over the time you have left before the test. Break your study plan into small, clear goals so you have a manageable task for each day and know exactly what you're doing. Then just focus on one small step at a time. When you manage your time this way, you don't need to spend hours at a time studying. Studying a small block of content for a short period each day helps you retain information better and avoid stressing over how much you have left to do. You can relax knowing that you have a plan to cover everything in time. In order for this strategy to be effective though, you have to start studying early and stick to your schedule. Avoid the exhaustion and futility that comes from last-minute cramming!

## Study Environment

The environment you study in has a big impact on your learning. Studying in a coffee shop, while probably more enjoyable, is not likely to be as fruitful as studying in a quiet room. It's important to keep distractions to a minimum. You're only planning to study for a short block of time, so make the most of it. Don't pause to check your phone or get up to find a snack. It's also important to **avoid multitasking**. Research has consistently shown that multitasking will make your studying dramatically less effective. Your study area should also be comfortable and well-lit so you don't have the distraction of straining your eyes or sitting on an uncomfortable chair.

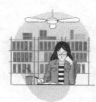 The time of day you study is also important. You want to be rested and alert. Don't wait until just before bedtime. Study when you'll be most likely to comprehend and remember. Even better, if you know what time of day your test will be, set that time aside for study. That way your brain will be used to working on that subject at that specific time and you'll have a better chance of recalling information.

Finally, it can be helpful to team up with others who are studying for the same test. Your actual studying should be done in as isolated an environment as possible, but the work of organizing the information and setting up the study plan can be divided up. In between study sessions, you can discuss with your teammates the concepts that you're all studying and quiz each other on the details. Just be sure that your teammates are as serious about the test as you are. If you find that your study time is being replaced with social time, you might need to find a new team.

# Secret Key #2 – Make Your Studying Count

You're devoting a lot of time and effort to preparing for this test, so you want to be absolutely certain it will pay off. This means doing more than just reading the content and hoping you can remember it on test day. It's important to make every minute of study count. There are two main areas you can focus on to make your studying count.

## Retention

It doesn't matter how much time you study if you can't remember the material. You need to make sure you are retaining the concepts. To check your retention of the information you're learning, try recalling it at later times with minimal prompting. Try carrying around flashcards and glance at one or two from time to time or ask a friend who's also studying for the test to quiz you.

To enhance your retention, look for ways to put the information into practice so that you can apply it rather than simply recalling it. If you're using the information in practical ways, it will be much easier to remember. Similarly, it helps to solidify a concept in your mind if you're not only reading it to yourself but also explaining it to someone else. Ask a friend to let you teach them about a concept you're a little shaky on (or speak aloud to an imaginary audience if necessary). As you try to summarize, define, give examples, and answer your friend's questions, you'll understand the concepts better and they will stay with you longer. Finally, step back for a big picture view and ask yourself how each piece of information fits with the whole subject. When you link the different concepts together and see them working together as a whole, it's easier to remember the individual components.

Finally, practice showing your work on any multi-step problems, even if you're just studying. Writing out each step you take to solve a problem will help solidify the process in your mind, and you'll be more likely to remember it during the test.

## Modality

*Modality* simply refers to the means or method by which you study. Choosing a study modality that fits your own individual learning style is crucial. No two people learn best in exactly the same way, so it's important to know your strengths and use them to your advantage.

For example, if you learn best by visualization, focus on visualizing a concept in your mind and draw an image or a diagram. Try color-coding your notes, illustrating them, or creating symbols that will trigger your mind to recall a learned concept. If you learn best by hearing or discussing information, find a study partner who learns the same way or read aloud to yourself. Think about how to put the information in your own words. Imagine that you are giving a lecture on the topic and record yourself so you can listen to it later.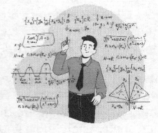

For any learning style, flashcards can be helpful. Organize the information so you can take advantage of spare moments to review. Underline key words or phrases. Use different colors for different categories. Mnemonic devices (such as creating a short list in which every item starts with the same letter) can also help with retention. Find what works best for you and use it to store the information in your mind most effectively and easily.

# Secret Key #3 – Practice the Right Way

Your success on test day depends not only on how many hours you put into preparing, but also on whether you prepared the right way. It's good to check along the way to see if your studying is paying off. One of the most effective ways to do this is by taking practice tests to evaluate your progress. Practice tests are useful because they show exactly where you need to improve. Every time you take a practice test, pay special attention to these three groups of questions:

- The questions you got wrong
- The questions you had to guess on, even if you guessed right
- The questions you found difficult or slow to work through

This will show you exactly what your weak areas are, and where you need to devote more study time. Ask yourself why each of these questions gave you trouble. Was it because you didn't understand the material? Was it because you didn't remember the vocabulary? Do you need more repetitions on this type of question to build speed and confidence? Dig into those questions and figure out how you can strengthen your weak areas as you go back to review the material.

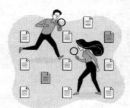 Additionally, many practice tests have a section explaining the answer choices. It can be tempting to read the explanation and think that you now have a good understanding of the concept. However, an explanation likely only covers part of the question's broader context. Even if the explanation makes perfect sense, **go back and investigate** every concept related to the question until you're positive you have a thorough understanding.

As you go along, keep in mind that the practice test is just that: practice. Memorizing these questions and answers will not be very helpful on the actual test because it is unlikely to have any of the same exact questions. If you only know the right answers to the sample questions, you won't be prepared for the real thing. **Study the concepts** until you understand them fully, and then you'll be able to answer any question that shows up on the test.

It's important to wait on the practice tests until you're ready. If you take a test on your first day of study, you may be overwhelmed by the amount of material covered and how much you need to learn. Work up to it gradually.

On test day, you'll need to be prepared for answering questions, managing your time, and using the test-taking strategies you've learned. It's a lot to balance, like a mental marathon that will have a big impact on your future. Like training for a marathon, you'll need to start slowly and work your way up. When test day arrives, you'll be ready.

Start with the strategies you've read in the first two Secret Keys—plan your course and study in the way that works best for you. If you have time, consider using multiple study resources to get different approaches to the same concepts. It can be helpful to see difficult concepts from more than one angle. Then find a good source for practice tests. Many times, the test website will suggest potential study resources or provide sample tests.

# Practice Test Strategy

If you're able to find at least three practice tests, we recommend this strategy:

### UNTIMED AND OPEN-BOOK PRACTICE

Take the first test with no time constraints and with your notes and study guide handy. Take your time and focus on applying the strategies you've learned.

### TIMED AND OPEN-BOOK PRACTICE

Take the second practice test open-book as well, but set a timer and practice pacing yourself to finish in time.

### TIMED AND CLOSED-BOOK PRACTICE

Take any other practice tests as if it were test day. Set a timer and put away your study materials. Sit at a table or desk in a quiet room, imagine yourself at the testing center, and answer questions as quickly and accurately as possible.

Keep repeating timed and closed-book tests on a regular basis until you run out of practice tests or it's time for the actual test. Your mind will be ready for the schedule and stress of test day, and you'll be able to focus on recalling the material you've learned.

# Secret Key #4 – Pace Yourself

Once you're fully prepared for the material on the test, your biggest challenge on test day will be managing your time. Just knowing that the clock is ticking can make you panic even if you have plenty of time left. Work on pacing yourself so you can build confidence against the time constraints of the exam. Pacing is a difficult skill to master, especially in a high-pressure environment, so **practice is vital**.

Set time expectations for your pace based on how much time is available. For example, if a section has 60 questions and the time limit is 30 minutes, you know you have to average 30 seconds or less per question in order to answer them all. Although 30 seconds is the hard limit, set 25 seconds per question as your goal, so you reserve extra time to spend on harder questions. When you budget extra time for the harder questions, you no longer have any reason to stress when those questions take longer to answer.

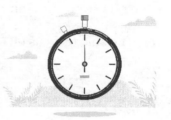

Don't let this time expectation distract you from working through the test at a calm, steady pace, but keep it in mind so you don't spend too much time on any one question. Recognize that taking extra time on one question you don't understand may keep you from answering two that you do understand later in the test. If your time limit for a question is up and you're still not sure of the answer, mark it and move on, and come back to it later if the time and the test format allow. If the testing format doesn't allow you to return to earlier questions, just make an educated guess; then put it out of your mind and move on.

On the easier questions, be careful not to rush. It may seem wise to hurry through them so you have more time for the challenging ones, but it's not worth missing one if you know the concept and just didn't take the time to read the question fully. Work efficiently but make sure you understand the question and have looked at all of the answer choices, since more than one may seem right at first.

Even if you're paying attention to the time, you may find yourself a little behind at some point. You should speed up to get back on track, but do so wisely. Don't panic; just take a few seconds less on each question until you're caught up. Don't guess without thinking, but do look through the answer choices and eliminate any you know are wrong. If you can get down to two choices, it is often worthwhile to guess from those. Once you've chosen an answer, move on and don't dwell on any that you skipped or had to hurry through. If a question was taking too long, chances are it was one of the harder ones, so you weren't as likely to get it right anyway.

On the other hand, if you find yourself getting ahead of schedule, it may be beneficial to slow down a little. The more quickly you work, the more likely you are to make a careless mistake that will affect your score. You've budgeted time for each question, so don't be afraid to spend that time. Practice an efficient but careful pace to get the most out of the time you have.

6

# Secret Key #5 – Have a Plan for Guessing

When you're taking the test, you may find yourself stuck on a question. Some of the answer choices seem better than others, but you don't see the one answer choice that is obviously correct. What do you do?

The scenario described above is very common, yet most test takers have not effectively prepared for it. Developing and practicing a plan for guessing may be one of the single most effective uses of your time as you get ready for the exam.

In developing your plan for guessing, there are three questions to address:

- When should you start the guessing process?
- How should you narrow down the choices?
- Which answer should you choose?

## When to Start the Guessing Process

Unless your plan for guessing is to select C every time (which, despite its merits, is not what we recommend), you need to leave yourself enough time to apply your answer elimination strategies. Since you have a limited amount of time for each question, that means that if you're going to give yourself the best shot at guessing correctly, you have to decide quickly whether or not you will guess.

Of course, the best-case scenario is that you don't have to guess at all, so first, see if you can answer the question based on your knowledge of the subject and basic reasoning skills. Focus on the key words in the question and try to jog your memory of related topics. Give yourself a chance to bring the knowledge to mind, but once you realize that you don't have (or you can't access) the knowledge you need to answer the question, it's time to start the guessing process.

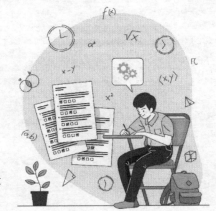

It's almost always better to start the guessing process too early than too late. It only takes a few seconds to remember something and answer the question from knowledge. Carefully eliminating wrong answer choices takes longer. Plus, going through the process of eliminating answer choices can actually help jog your memory.

**Summary**: Start the guessing process as soon as you decide that you can't answer the question based on your knowledge.

# How to Narrow Down the Choices

The next chapter in this book (**Test-Taking Strategies**) includes a wide range of strategies for how to approach questions and how to look for answer choices to eliminate. You will definitely want to read those carefully, practice them, and figure out which ones work best for you. Here though, we're going to address a mindset rather than a particular strategy.

Your odds of guessing an answer correctly depend on how many options you are choosing from.

| Number of options left | 5 | 4 | 3 | 2 | 1 |
| --- | --- | --- | --- | --- | --- |
| Odds of guessing correctly | 20% | 25% | 33% | 50% | 100% |

You can see from this chart just how valuable it is to be able to eliminate incorrect answers and make an educated guess, but there are two things that many test takers do that cause them to miss out on the benefits of guessing:

- Accidentally eliminating the correct answer
- Selecting an answer based on an impression

We'll look at the first one here, and the second one in the next section.

To avoid accidentally eliminating the correct answer, we recommend a thought exercise called **the $5 challenge**. In this challenge, you only eliminate an answer choice from contention if you are willing to bet $5 on it being wrong. Why $5? Five dollars is a small but not insignificant amount of money. It's an amount you could afford to lose but wouldn't want to throw away. And while losing

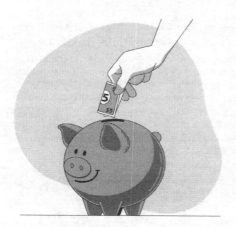

$5 once might not hurt too much, doing it twenty times will set you back $100. In the same way, each small decision you make—eliminating a choice here, guessing on a question there—won't by itself impact your score very much, but when you put them all together, they can make a big difference. By holding each answer choice elimination decision to a higher standard, you can reduce the risk of accidentally eliminating the correct answer.

The $5 challenge can also be applied in a positive sense: If you are willing to bet $5 that an answer choice *is* correct, go ahead and mark it as correct.

**Summary**: Only eliminate an answer choice if you are willing to bet $5 that it is wrong.

8

# Which Answer to Choose

You're taking the test. You've run into a hard question and decided you'll have to guess. You've eliminated all the answer choices you're willing to bet $5 on. Now you have to pick an answer. Why do we even need to talk about this? Why can't you just pick whichever one you feel like when the time comes?

The answer to these questions is that if you don't come into the test with a plan, you'll rely on your impression to select an answer choice, and if you do that, you risk falling into a trap. The test writers know that everyone who takes their test will be guessing on some of the questions, so they intentionally write wrong answer choices to seem plausible. You still have to pick an answer though, and if the wrong answer choices are designed to look right, how can you ever be sure that you're not falling for their trap? The best solution we've found to this dilemma is to take the decision out of your hands entirely. Here is the process we recommend:

**Once you've eliminated any choices that you are confident (willing to bet $5) are wrong, select the first remaining choice as your answer.**

Whether you choose to select the first remaining choice, the second, or the last, the important thing is that you use some preselected standard. Using this approach guarantees that you will not be enticed into selecting an answer choice that looks right, because you are not basing your decision on how the answer choices look.

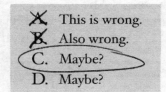

This is not meant to make you question your knowledge. Instead, it is to help you recognize the difference between your knowledge and your impressions. There's a huge difference between thinking an answer is right because of what you know, and thinking an answer is right because it looks or sounds like it should be right.

**Summary**: To ensure that your selection is appropriately random, make a predetermined selection from among all answer choices you have not eliminated.

# Test-Taking Strategies

This section contains a list of test-taking strategies that you may find helpful as you work through the test. By taking what you know and applying logical thought, you can maximize your chances of answering any question correctly!

It is very important to realize that every question is different and every person is different: no single strategy will work on every question, and no single strategy will work for every person. That's why we've included all of them here, so you can try them out and determine which ones work best for different types of questions and which ones work best for you.

## Question Strategies

### ☑ READ CAREFULLY

Read the question and the answer choices carefully. Don't miss the question because you misread the terms. You have plenty of time to read each question thoroughly and make sure you understand what is being asked. Yet a happy medium must be attained, so don't waste too much time. You must read carefully and efficiently.

### ☑ CONTEXTUAL CLUES

Look for contextual clues. If the question includes a word you are not familiar with, look at the immediate context for some indication of what the word might mean. Contextual clues can often give you all the information you need to decipher the meaning of an unfamiliar word. Even if you can't determine the meaning, you may be able to narrow down the possibilities enough to make a solid guess at the answer to the question.

### ☑ PREFIXES

If you're having trouble with a word in the question or answer choices, try dissecting it. Take advantage of every clue that the word might include. Prefixes can be a huge help. Usually, they allow you to determine a basic meaning. *Pre-* means before, *post-* means after, *pro-* is positive, *de-* is negative. From prefixes, you can get an idea of the general meaning of the word and try to put it into context.

### ☑ HEDGE WORDS

Watch out for critical hedge words, such as *likely, may, can, sometimes, often, almost, mostly, usually, generally, rarely,* and *sometimes.* Question writers insert these hedge phrases to cover every possibility. Often an answer choice will be wrong simply because it leaves no room for exception. Be on guard for answer choices that have definitive words such as *exactly* and *always*.

### ☑ SWITCHBACK WORDS

Stay alert for *switchbacks*. These are the words and phrases frequently used to alert you to shifts in thought. The most common switchback words are *but, although,* and *however.* Others include *nevertheless, on the other hand, even though, while, in spite of, despite,* and *regardless of.* Switchback words are important to catch because they can change the direction of the question or an answer choice.

10

### ☑ FACE VALUE

When in doubt, use common sense. Accept the situation in the problem at face value. Don't read too much into it. These problems will not require you to make wild assumptions. If you have to go beyond creativity and warp time or space in order to have an answer choice fit the question, then you should move on and consider the other answer choices. These are normal problems rooted in reality. The applicable relationship or explanation may not be readily apparent, but it is there for you to figure out. Use your common sense to interpret anything that isn't clear.

## Answer Choice Strategies

### ☑ ANSWER SELECTION

The most thorough way to pick an answer choice is to identify and eliminate wrong answers until only one is left, then confirm it is the correct answer. Sometimes an answer choice may immediately seem right, but be careful. The test writers will usually put more than one reasonable answer choice on each question, so take a second to read all of them and make sure that the other choices are not equally obvious. As long as you have time left, it is better to read every answer choice than to pick the first one that looks right without checking the others.

### ☑ ANSWER CHOICE FAMILIES

An answer choice family consists of two (in rare cases, three) answer choices that are very similar in construction and cannot all be true at the same time. If you see two answer choices that are direct opposites or parallels, one of them is usually the correct answer. For instance, if one answer choice says that quantity $x$ increases and another either says that quantity $x$ decreases (opposite) or says that quantity $y$ increases (parallel), then those answer choices would fall into the same family. An answer choice that doesn't match the construction of the answer choice family is more likely to be incorrect. Most questions will not have answer choice families, but when they do appear, you should be prepared to recognize them.

### ☑ ELIMINATE ANSWERS

Eliminate answer choices as soon as you realize they are wrong, but make sure you consider all possibilities. If you are eliminating answer choices and realize that the last one you are left with is also wrong, don't panic. Start over and consider each choice again. There may be something you missed the first time that you will realize on the second pass.

### ☑ AVOID FACT TRAPS

Don't be distracted by an answer choice that is factually true but doesn't answer the question. You are looking for the choice that answers the question. Stay focused on what the question is asking for so you don't accidentally pick an answer that is true but incorrect. Always go back to the question and make sure the answer choice you've selected actually answers the question and is not merely a true statement.

### ☑ EXTREME STATEMENTS

In general, you should avoid answers that put forth extreme actions as standard practice or proclaim controversial ideas as established fact. An answer choice that states the "process should be used in certain situations, if..." is much more likely to be correct than one that states the "process should be discontinued completely." The first is a calm rational statement and doesn't even make a definitive, uncompromising stance, using a hedge word *if* to provide wiggle room, whereas the second choice is far more extreme.

### ⊘ BENCHMARK

As you read through the answer choices and you come across one that seems to answer the question well, mentally select that answer choice. This is not your final answer, but it's the one that will help you evaluate the other answer choices. The one that you selected is your benchmark or standard for judging each of the other answer choices. Every other answer choice must be compared to your benchmark. That choice is correct until proven otherwise by another answer choice beating it. If you find a better answer, then that one becomes your new benchmark. Once you've decided that no other choice answers the question as well as your benchmark, you have your final answer.

### ⊘ PREDICT THE ANSWER

Before you even start looking at the answer choices, it is often best to try to predict the answer. When you come up with the answer on your own, it is easier to avoid distractions and traps because you will know exactly what to look for. The right answer choice is unlikely to be word-for-word what you came up with, but it should be a close match. Even if you are confident that you have the right answer, you should still take the time to read each option before moving on.

## General Strategies

### ⊘ TOUGH QUESTIONS

If you are stumped on a problem or it appears too hard or too difficult, don't waste time. Move on! Remember though, if you can quickly check for obviously incorrect answer choices, your chances of guessing correctly are greatly improved. Before you completely give up, at least try to knock out a couple of possible answers. Eliminate what you can and then guess at the remaining answer choices before moving on.

### ⊘ CHECK YOUR WORK

Since you will probably not know every term listed and the answer to every question, it is important that you get credit for the ones that you do know. Don't miss any questions through careless mistakes. If at all possible, try to take a second to look back over your answer selection and make sure you've selected the correct answer choice and haven't made a costly careless mistake (such as marking an answer choice that you didn't mean to mark). This quick double check should more than pay for itself in caught mistakes for the time it costs.

### ⊘ PACE YOURSELF

It's easy to be overwhelmed when you're looking at a page full of questions; your mind is confused and full of random thoughts, and the clock is ticking down faster than you would like. Calm down and maintain the pace that you have set for yourself. Especially as you get down to the last few minutes of the test, don't let the small numbers on the clock make you panic. As long as you are on track by monitoring your pace, you are guaranteed to have time for each question.

### ⊘ DON'T RUSH

It is very easy to make errors when you are in a hurry. Maintaining a fast pace in answering questions is pointless if it makes you miss questions that you would have gotten right otherwise. Test writers like to include distracting information and wrong answers that seem right. Taking a little extra time to avoid careless mistakes can make all the difference in your test score. Find a pace that allows you to be confident in the answers that you select.

## ⊘ Keep Moving

Panicking will not help you pass the test, so do your best to stay calm and keep moving. Taking deep breaths and going through the answer elimination steps you practiced can help to break through a stress barrier and keep your pace.

# Final Notes

The combination of a solid foundation of content knowledge and the confidence that comes from practicing your plan for applying that knowledge is the key to maximizing your performance on test day. As your foundation of content knowledge is built up and strengthened, you'll find that the strategies included in this chapter become more and more effective in helping you quickly sift through the distractions and traps of the test to isolate the correct answer.

Now that you're preparing to move forward into the test content chapters of this book, be sure to keep your goal in mind. As you read, think about how you will be able to apply this information on the test. If you've already seen sample questions for the test and you have an idea of the question format and style, try to come up with questions of your own that you can answer based on what you're reading. This will give you valuable practice applying your knowledge in the same ways you can expect to on test day.

**Good luck and good studying!**

# Evaluation and Assessment

## STAGES OF FETAL DEVELOPMENT

The three stages of **fetal development** are the **germinal phase**, the **embryonic phase**, and the **fetal stage**. The germinal phase begins at the point of conception when the sperm meets the egg and continues for 2 weeks. The outer cells form the placenta, and the inner cells will form the embryo. The cells continue to divide, and a blastocyst is formed. The embryonic phase begins 3 to 8 weeks after conception when the embryo implants in the uterus. During this time, the neural tube is formed, and it will eventually become the central nervous system, spine, and brain. The forebrain, midbrain, and hindbrain are created from ridges in the neural tube. The head and its structures (eyes, ears, nose, and mouth) are formed, the heart begins to beat, arm and leg buds appear, and the central and peripheral nervous system and brain are recognizable. The fetal stage is 9 weeks post conception to birth. During this phase, the brain and spinal cord began to fully form from the neural tube; reflexes emerge and genitals appear; nails, eyelashes, tooth buds and hair appear; and lungs fully develop.

## BLASTOCYST

As the embryo divides and travels to the uterus, a **blastocyst** is formed. The blastocyst has three distinct layers from which all major organ systems will be formed. The outermost layer of the blastocyst forms the trophoblast, which will become the placenta. The innermost layers of the blastocyst will form the ectoderm, endoderm, and mesoderm. The outer layer is the ectoderm. This layer will form the hair, skin, nails, and nervous system. The middle layer is the endoderm, and it will form the respiratory and digestive systems. The inner layer is the mesoderm, and it will form the skeleton and muscles.

## SCREENING FOR AND IDENTIFYING BIRTH DEFECTS

New moms will often opt to screen for birth defects during pregnancy to provide time to make tough decisions and get resources in place prior to birth. During the first trimester, blood work can show if a fetus is predisposed to or at a higher risk for neural tube defects, heart defects, and chromosomal disorders such as **Down syndrome**. Down syndrome is a genetic disorder caused when abnormal cell division results in extra genetic material from chromosome 21. During the second trimester, an ultrasound can identify a cleft palate or structural issues of limbs and organs, and a **fetal nuchal translucency (NT)** exam looks for excess fluid buildup at the base of the neck under the skin, which can again indicate Down syndrome, heart defects, and many chromosomal defects. A blood test in the second trimester can show if there is an excess of protein, which can indicate an open neural tube, Down syndrome, or a chromosomal defect. If blood work in the early trimesters indicates abnormalities or puts the mother at high risk, an amniocentesis can be performed between weeks 15 and 20. In this procedure, amniotic fluid is extracted and sent to the lab. This will bring the most specific results identifying chromosomal defects and neural tube defects. Many women opt not to have this test because of the risk of preterm labor, maternal infection, and miscarriage.

## CORRECTED AGE IN PREMATURE BABIES

A corrected age is used for babies that are born prematurely. This becomes important to monitor and assess if the baby is hitting milestones, and it allows providers to evaluate his or her abilities compared to other children the same age. A **chronological age** or actual age is how old the child is from the date of delivery. This is their birthday. A **corrected age** adjusts for the prematurity level of the child. Therapists will likely use the corrected age until the child is 3 years old. At that time, the

Copyright © Mometrix Media. You have been licensed one copy of this document for personal use only. Any other reproduction or redistribution is strictly prohibited. All rights reserved.
This content is provided for test preparation purposes only and does not imply an endorsement by Mometrix of any particular political, scientific, or religious point of view.

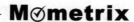

child has usually caught up to the abilities of a child that was born full term. The formula to calculate this is as follows: **(chronological age) – (weeks or months of prematurity) = corrected age.** If the baby is born at 28 weeks, he is 12 weeks premature. If the baby has a chronological age of 6 months old, (6 months) – (3 months) = (3 months).

## PRIMITIVE REFLEXES IN NEWBORNS

A **primitive reflex** is an involuntary reaction to a stimulus. Reflexes develop in utero and become integrated as we age. If a primitive reflex has not integrated and disappeared by a certain age, that is often seen as a sign of a neurological issue or brain damage. There are seven primitive reflexes seen in a newborn. The Moro, rooting, and palmar reflexes are explained as follows:

| Reflex | Characteristics | Integrated |
|---|---|---|
| Moro | Early fight-or-flight reflex. It is stimulated by a sudden lack of support when the baby feels as though it is falling. This is tested by holding the torso and head of the baby off the exam table and then letting the head and shoulders drop quickly several inches. The baby will look startled, extend its arms and legs out, bring them back in, and cry. | 3 months |
| Rooting | Present even before birth. When the baby is stimulated by a touch to the cheek on either side, the baby will turn his head to that direction in preparation to suck. This reflex is integrated by 4 months. | 4 months |
| Palmar | This is caused when the baby's palm is stimulated. The baby will make a fist and grasp the object, and the fist will tighten as you try to remove the object. | 6 months |

## TYPES OF NEURAL TUBE DEFECTS

There are two types of **neural tube defects (NTDs)**: **open** and **closed**. These occur in the first month of pregnancy when the embryonic phase occurs. The neural tube forms against the neural plate in an embryo. Two ridges form, and as they close, a tube develops and vesicles are created. These become the vesicles of the brain that become the forebrain, midbrain, and hindbrain. An open NTD is when the tube does not fully close and portions of the brain or spinal cord are open to the environment. In a closed NTD, the defect is covered by skin. The most common of these defects is **spina bifida**, which usually causes paralysis below the level of where the tube has failed and not closed. Babies born with this diagnosis will likely have ambulation or mobility deficits as well as bowel and bladder issues because these areas are affected by the most distal spinal nerves.

## LESS-COMMON OPEN NEURAL TUBE DEFECTS

Three open neural tube defects (NTDs) that are less common are **anencephaly**, **encephalocele**, and **iniencephaly**. Anencephaly is caused when the area at the top of the tube does not close. The fetus will have little brain matter, and they are typically born deaf, blind, paralyzed, and will often not live long after birth if not stillborn. Encephalocele is when the tube fails near the brain and the brain pushes out the opening. This can cause developmental delays, paralysis or ataxic movement, seizures, and deformities of the head and face. Iniencephaly is when the spine is malformed causing the head to bend back at a severe angle giving the appearance of no neck. Cleft lip and palate are common, as are cardiac issues. Again, in this defect, death is shortly after birth.

## POSITIONAL PRIMITIVE REFLEXES

The positional primitive reflexes are as follows:

- **Plantar/Babinski reflex**: The bottom of the foot is stroked firmly moving from the heel to the toes. The big toe bends back toward the foot, and the toes splay out. Integrated at 2 years
- **Asymmetrical tonic neck reflex**: This is known as the fencing reflex. When the baby is on his back and his head is turned to one side, the arm and leg extend in the direction that the baby is facing and the other arm and leg flex. Integrated at 3 months
- **Spinal Galant reflex**: The baby is on her stomach and is stimulated firmly on one side of her spine in a downward motion. The hips will laterally flex toward the stimulus. This is thought to assist in rolling and crawling. Integrated at 9 months
- **Symmetrical tonic neck reflex**: The chin of the baby is tipped to his chest. The arms flex, and the legs will extend. Present at birth then disappears and returns at 6 months being integrated by 11 months to 1 year.

## MOTOR DEVELOPMENT

### VOLUNTARY REACH AND GRASP

The first signs of voluntary grasp and release is seen at 4 months old. Initially the child will see an object he desires and reach with for it with one hand. When the child sees that he has made contact with the item, the hand will grasp and close. As he matures, he will use two hands to reach using his vision to target the item, and the action of grasping is stimulated by touch versus vision. Reaching develops from a sweeping movement of the hand and arm in a backhanded motion toward the object to a scooping movement transitioning to a direct reach. In a mature grasp, the parts of the reach grasp process are (1) locating the object (visual regard), (2) reaching the object (postural control and arm movement), (3) grasping the object (grip pattern), and (4) manipulation.

### POSTURAL CONTROL IN A CHILD DURING THE FIRST YEAR

**Postural control** is the ability to maintain the body in an upright position without support. In the first year of life, postural control begins with the ability to hold the head up independently. The next step is trunk control in sitting. This is followed by transitioning from a seated position to quadruped. From quadruped, a child moves into standing and then to walking and running.

| Prone development | Weight-bearing from torso, lifts head with weight-bearing in lower extremities, weight-bearing through forearms and hands, weight-bearing in hands with elbows extended rolling prone to supine, and quadruped rocking. |
| --- | --- |
| Supine development | The head can't stay at midline and drops to either side, the head can be held neutral with neck flexion and the baby can get hands to mouth, can hold things at midline playing and grabbing at feet and can lay on his side, and can roll to prone without rotating hips first. |
| Quadruped development | Rounded spine and can't sit without support, can bear weight in quadruped and scoot in reverse, move in and out of an unsupported sitting position, and creeps. |
| Standing development | Stepping reflex when being held vertically, partial weight-bearing when in a supported stand, pulls to stand and furniture cruising, can take steps with hand holding, and walks independently. |

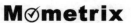

## FINE MOTOR DEVELOPMENT TIMELINE

**Fine motor skills** develop from experience and practice. These skills usually involve dexterity, hand-eye coordination, manipulation, and finger strength. The best way to encourage fine motor skills is playing with toys such as Legos or stringing beads or arts and crafts.

| Age | Skill |
|---|---|
| 3 months | Bilateral palmar grasp |
| 6 months | Holds and brings hands together |
| 9 months | Transfers objects between hands, accurate reaching |
| 12 months | Pincer grasp, controlled release |
| 2 years | Scribbles, self-feeds, turns pages |
| 3 years | Hand dominance, snips with scissors, tripod grasp |
| 4 years | Copies shapes, stabilizes objects with nondominant hand |
| 5 years | Cuts on line, dresses independently, writes name |

## CHILD DEVELOPMENT MILESTONES FROM 2 MONTHS TO 5 YEARS

**Child development milestones** are the functional skills and traits seen in children as they develop. Milestones are used to determine if a child is developing typically or if there is reason for concern.

| Age | Milestone |
|---|---|
| 2 months | Self-soothes, turns head to find noises, begins to track objects, and can lift head during tummy time |
| 4 months | Begins to smile and babble, can reach for a toy or desired object, and can push himself to his elbows during tummy time. |
| 6 months | Responds to her name, identifies familiar faces, brings things to her mouth, sits without support, can rock in quadruped for precrawling. |
| 9 months | Can transition toys between hands crossing the midline, uses a pincer grip to pick up small items, "stranger danger" emerges, crawls, pulls to standing, points at things he desires, and will imitate sounds and gestures. |
| 12 months | Begins to help with dressing, cries when parents leave, uses simple words, begins to feed with utensils, follows simple one-step commands, walking, and "cruising." |
| 18 months | Temper tantrums, pretend play, drinking from a cup, knows simple body parts, uses a fisting grip to scribble. |
| 2 years | Two- to four-word sentences, knows names of familiar people and items, hand dominance emerges, flows two-step commands consistently, can run, walk upstairs, throw a ball, jump with two feet, knows colors and basic animals, and can repeat words heard during conversations. |
| 3 years | Follows three-step commands, turn-taking, fine motor skills mature, buttons and zippers become easier, climbs, copies circles and lines, and begins to identify her name and age. |
| 4 years | Plays house and make-believe, begins counting, can draw a person with four body parts, uses scissors, can hop on one foot, and can bounce and kick a ball consistently. |
| 5 years | Speaks clearly and uses full sentences, copies more complex shapes, skips and swings, can use the bathroom on his own, and wants to be like his friends. |

## SELF-CARE EMERGENCE FROM BIRTH TO AGE 6

Self-care tasks or **activities of daily living (ADLs)** are activities that include dressing, bathing, toileting and eating, transferring, hygiene, and grooming.

| Age | Activities |
|---|---|
| 3 months | Communicates needs through crying |
| 6 months | Self-feeds small items |
| 9 months | Holds cup independently, tolerates a variety of food textures |
| 12 months | Brushes teeth and removes socks, shoes, and pants |
| 2 years | Toileting with assistance, able to use large buttons and snaps |
| 3 years | Using a napkin, toileting independently, using utensils consistently |
| 4 years | Choosing clothing and dressing independently |
| 5 years | Packing a bag for school, using zipper-top bags and lunch box items independently |
| 6 years | Making simple meals, bathing independently |

## TIMELINE AND ACTIVITIES ENCOURAGING GROSS MOTOR DEVELOPMENT

**Gross motor skills** develop from the torso and move to the extremities. They also move from the top of the body distally. There are three categories of gross motor skills. **Stability**, **locomotive**, and **manipulative**. Stability skills involve weight shifting and balance. Locomotive involve moving the body physically in space. This could be crawling, rolling, walking, and running. Manipulative involves moving an object between hands or through space such as throwing a ball or jumping rope.

| Age | Skill |
|---|---|
| 3 months | Hold head up |
| 6 months | Can roll front to back |
| 9 months | Sit and crawl |
| 12 months | Walk |
| 2 years | Run |
| 3 years | Climb, jump, kick |
| 4 years | Ride a tricycle/bike |
| 5 years | Skip, balance on one foot, gallop |

The best way to encourage gross motor skills is by play through tumbling, roughhousing, dance, sports, obstacle courses, and games such as Simon says.

## CLASSIFICATIONS OF GENERAL GRASP PATTERNS

Grasp patterns are the movements of the hand used to pick up and hold objects in daily life. Hand movements can be **prehensile** and **nonprehensile**. Prehensile can be a precision movement (using the thumb in opposition to the fingers) or a power movement (using the whole hand).

- **Hook:** The fingers hook around an object. Seen when carrying a briefcase.
- **Power:** A category of cylindrical grasp used when force is needed and the thumb stabilizes. Gripping a hairbrush or hammer.
- **Lateral pinch:** When the thumb acts as a stabilizer against the index finger. This is when you are using a key.
- **Pincer (pad-to-pad/two-point pinch):** The thumb and pointer fingertips meet. This is used to pick up small items such as Cheerios.
- **Cylindrical grasp:** Holding a baseball bat or soda can. The thumb is flexed and abducted while the fingers encircle the object.

- **Spherical grasp:** This is when the whole hand wraps around the object with the thumb in opposition, for example, holding a baseball.
- **Three-jaw chuck (three-point pincer):** Stacking small blocks. The index and middle fingers are flexed with an opposed thumb, and the ring and little fingers stabilize from the ulnar side.

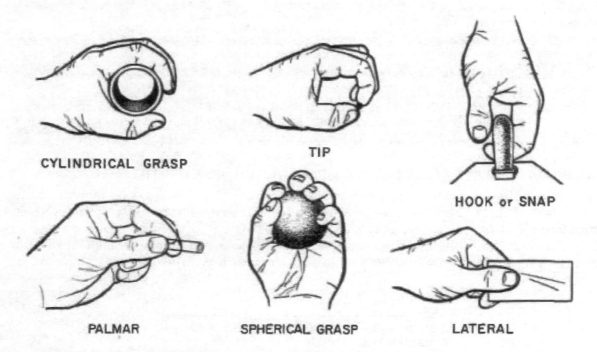

CYLINDRICAL GRASP        TIP        HOOK or SNAP

PALMAR        SPHERICAL GRASP        LATERAL

## PATTERNS AND PROCESS OF IN-HAND MANIPULATION SKILLS

**In-hand manipulation** is the ability to hold and move an object within one hand. This skill can be broken down into three parts: **translation**, **shift**, and **rotation**. Translation is the ability to move objects from the fingertips to the palm or the palm to the fingertips. Shift is the ability to move an object in a linear pattern with the fingertips. Rotation is the ability to turn an object around in the pads of the fingers and thumb. There are five patterns to in-hand manipulation:

| Pattern | Examples |
|---|---|
| Finger to palm | Getting change out of a change purse or picking up multiple utensils at one time when setting the table. |
| Palm to finger | Playing a game such as Connect Four. Moving the disc piece from the palm to the finger to place in the slot. |
| Shift | Adjusting the pencil when you pick it up so that your grip is at the tip of the pencil or moving keys on a key ring to find the correct key. |
| Simple rotation | Unscrewing the cap of a water bottle or rotating a puzzle piece. |
| Complex rotation | Flipping a pencil over to use the eraser or rotating two objects in the hand at the same time. |

## DEVELOPMENT OF PREWRITING SKILLS IN CHILDREN

Prewriting skills are the ability for children to create straight lines, curved lines, zigzags, and shapes in order to build the foundation for letter and number formation.

| Age | Skill |
| --- | --- |
| 10–12 months | Scribbles on paper with no specific goals. Random and spontaneous. |
| 2 years | Can imitate horizontal and vertical lines as well as curved and circular shapes. |
| 3 years | Can copy horizontal and vertical lines in addition to circles. |
| 4–5 years | Can copy simple letters and numbers; copy or trace name; copy a cross shape, right and left diagonal lines, and a square; and can imitate an X shape. |
| 5–6 years | Can print his own name, copy a triangle, and copy the upper- and lowercase letters of the alphabet. |

## TYPES OF THE MATURE PENCIL GRASP

A **mature pencil grasp** is when a child can write legibly, without fatigue, and at a pace that is reasonable. Types of the mature pencil grasps:

- **Radial cross-palmar** (Age 0–2): The pencil is positioned across the palm held with a fisted hand with the thumb toward the paper.
- **Palmar supinate** (Age 1–2): The pencil is positioned across the palm held with a fisted hand with the little finger toward the paper.
- **Digital pronate** (Age 2–3): The fingers hold the pencil, and the palm faces down toward the page with the index finger used for stability.
- **Brush** (Age 2–3): The pencil is held with all the fingers with the top of the pencil positioned against palm. The hand is in prone position, and the whole arm and wrist create the movement.
- **Extended fingers** (Age 2–4): The pencil is held with all of the fingers. The wrist is straight and in the prone position with ulnar deviation, and the entire forearm moves. There is no isolated finger movement.
- **Four fingers** (Age 3–4): Four fingers are holding the pencil with the little finger stabilizing the paper forming a large space between the thumb and index finger.
- **Cross-thumb grasp** (Age 4–6): The fingers are curled into the palm, and the pencil rests against the index finger with the thumb crossed over the pencil toward the index finger. The fingers and wrist move, and the forearm stabilizes against the writing surface.
- **Static tripod** (Age 4–6): A three-finger grasp in which the thumb, index, and middle fingers work together as one unit and the top of the pencil rests on the metacarpophalangeal (MCP) joint.
- **Lateral tripod** (Age 5–7): The index finger is on top of the pencil with the thumb across the index finger between the proximal interphalangeal (PIP) and distal interphalangeal (DIP) joints.
- **Dynamic tripod** (Age 5–7): This pencil is held by the thumb, index, and middle fingers, which move independently from the ring and little fingers. The web space is open and becomes circular with the pencil resting across the web space.

## KEY PARTS OF A PEDIATRIC EVALUATION

The main parts of a **pediatric evaluation** are the background and developmental information, the caregiver interview, observation and standardized testing, evaluation, and the summary report. In the background and developmental part of the evaluation, medical charts are reviewed. Information on birth complications, developmental history, and Individualized Education Programs

(IEPs) and any previous reports from other providers, educators, or previous interventions are examined. During the caregiver interview, information comes directly from the parent or guardian. Concerns are raised about abilities, behaviors, habits, self-care, gross and fine motor skills, social skills, and play skills. During the interview, the parent can identify goals that they would like the child to achieve through therapy. All of this information will help the therapist determine what standardized tests are most appropriate to determine the areas of concern. In the observation and standardized testing portion of the evaluation, the therapist will spend time playing with and building rapport with the child. During this time, observations will be made on the integration of reflexes, fine and gross motor skills, motor planning, sensory processing skills, ADLs ability, behaviors, self-regulation, play skills, interaction, and attachment issues. The summary report is just as it sounds. In this piece, the therapist will summarize all the information gathered in the previous sections, make clinical judgments based on observations and testing, identify deficits and concerns, create goals, and establish a treatment length.

## MASLOW'S HIERARCHY OF NEEDS

**Maslow's hierarchy of needs** is a motivational psychological theory created in the 1940s based on the idea that a human being will be more successful as their basic needs are met. This is represented by placing each of the five concepts in the form of a pyramid with the base being the most basic need and the apex being self-actualization.

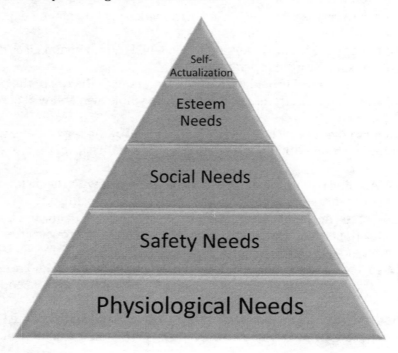

Maslow's five concepts are:

| Concept | Description |
| --- | --- |
| Self-actualization | This can be different for each person. Self-actualization comes from having your basic needs met and discovering what is important to you. At this level you determine if you are creating a life in which you are living up to your potential and meeting the goals you have set for yourself. |
| Esteem | This can be seen in two parts: (1) Do you have respect from others, friends, peers, at work, in the community? (2) Do you feel like you are contributing to life and that what you do matters in the bigger picture? |

22

| Concept | Description |
|---|---|
| Social | Humans need friends or family that they can connect with on an emotional and deep level. Do you have a community that you belong to, and will the members be there for you if you need them? This is unconditional acceptance. |
| Safety | People need a place to feel safe to move to the next level. This is about physical safety and avoiding violence. Are you fearful of something constantly, or do you feel free from harm? Do you have a safe place to sleep at night, or are you sleeping in the street? Are you being bullied? |
| Physiological | These are the most basic needs that we can't survive without: food, water, sleep, and shelter. |

## PIAGET'S STAGES OF INTELLECTUAL DEVELOPMENT

The four stages of intellectual development are the sensorimotor stage, preoperational stage, concrete operational stage, and the formal operational stage. The **sensorimotor stage** is birth to 2 years old. Everything the child learns in this stage comes from sensory input: touch, taste, feel, hear, and smell. Motor response to sensory input begins to develop, and object permanence becomes real as they learn that things exist even when they are not seen. The **preoperational stage** is between the ages of 2 and 7. During this time, a child begins to communicate with symbols, pictures, and words to represent different objects. Thinking is concrete and absolute, and the child is egocentric, not having the ability to empathize or understand that someone else may have a different perspective. The **concrete operational stage** is from age 7 to 11 years old. In this stage, children begin to think more in a more organized and logical way, but still concretely. They enjoy following rules in school. Abstract terms and ideas are not yet understood. They begin to realize that they have unique thoughts and that not everyone has the same thoughts and feelings as they do. They are able to start using inductive reasoning, moving from specific to general topics in conversations and activities. The **formal operational stage** is from age 11 and older. In this stage, children begin to think about abstract concepts, using deductive reasoning and seeing moral and ethical ramifications to their actions.

## ERIKSON'S STAGES OF PSYCHOSOCIAL DEVELOPMENT

**Erikson's psychosocial development theory** states that two opposing ideas must become resolved in order to become a productive member of society.

- **Stage 1**: Trust vs. Mistrust (Age 0-1.5)

  The world is uncertain and you look to your primary caregiver for consistency and stability. Success Virtue: Hope

- **Stage 2**: Autonomy vs. Shame (Age 1.5-3)

  Letting a child explore while being encouraging of success and tolerant in failure. Success Virtue: Will

- **Stage 3**: Initiative vs. Guilt (Age 3-5)

  Children assert their power by directing play and making their own decisions. They need to explore their abilities while parents encourage good choices by modeling good behavior. Success Virtue: Purpose

- **Stage 4**: Industry vs. Inferiority (Age 5-12)

Children feel the need to seek approval by being good at things deemed important in society like reading, math and physical abilities. Parents need to offer encouragement and not associate success in these areas with love.
Success Virtue: Competency

- **Stage 5**: Identity vs. Role Confusion (Age 12-18)

  Children begin to experiment with different identities, style, activities to discover who they want to be. Parents should encourage them and support their seeking nature to discover who they are.
  Success Virtue: Fidelity

- **Stage 6**: Intimacy vs. Isolation (Age 18-40)

  The goal is to find intimate and loving companionship and relationships. A poor sense of self will make this difficult to achieve.
  Success Virtue: Love

- **Stage 7**: Generativity vs. Stagnation (Age 40-65)

  Finding a way to make your mark or impact on the world. Failure in this area will feel like being an unproductive member in society.
  Success Virtue: Care

- **Stage 8**: Ego Integrity vs. Despair (Age 65+)

  This is triggered by major life events, losing a loved one, retirement, illness. Failure in this area leads to the questions "Did I live a meaningful life?" Do you have regrets or are you happy with your life?
  Success Virtue: Wisdom

## STAGES OF SOCIAL PLAY

There are six stages of social play. The first three of these are unoccupied play, solitary play, and onlooker play. **Unoccupied play** is from birth to 2 years old. This is when a child is focused on what they are doing, and it appears to be random movements with no specific purpose. The child is getting to know the environment and how they can move in it. **Solitary play** is from 2 to 3 years old. During this time, a child will be content to play alone and focus intently on the item they are playing with for long stretches of time. They will often not pay attention to other people or activities going on around them; this is how they learn to entertain themselves. **Onlooker play** is between 3 to 4 years old. This is when a child will watch others play but will not participate in the activity themselves. They will often talk to the other children playing about the activity or the rules of the game, but they will not play and join in the activity.

The last three stages of social play development are **parallel play**, **associative play**, and **cooperative play**. Parallel play can be between 2 and 4 years old. In this stage of play, children will often be playing with the same toy or activity but not together. They are playing near each other or even side by side but not interacting with each other. They are learning from each other but not engaging each other. Associative play is from age 3 into preschool and early kindergarten. Children will play together but will not have a common goal for their activity. The focus moves from the toys themselves to a focus on the other children. They engage and talk and even share toys, but they do not set rules or restrictions on their activities. Cooperative play occurs at ages 4 to 6. Children begin to organize and play together using specific rules and using teamwork. Activities will often have a

24

leader and set jobs for other players. The focus becomes the other children and the task at hand. Cooperative play is the culmination and the melding of all the previous types of play.

## AGE RANGES AND DEVELOPMENTAL TASKS OF EARLY, MIDDLE, AND LATE ADULTHOOD

Young adulthood is 20 to 40 years of age. The developmental tasks include the following: becoming an independent person; creating your own identity including style, likes, and dislikes, preferences and beliefs; creating a home of your own; establishing a career; acknowledging parents' limitations; establishing intimate relationships with friends and a mate; and raising children. Middle adulthood ranges from 40 to 65 years of age. The developmental tasks include: helping your children begin their own life and becoming empty nesters, death of parents, developing new leisure activities, midlife crises or sudden change of career paths, accepting physical and social changes that come with middle age, developing a social conscience, and creating a legacy. Late adulthood ranges from 65 and older. The developmental tasks include: aging in place, physical and mental changes, loss of a spouse and peers, acknowledging one's own mortality, retirement and fixed incomes, and becoming grandparents.

## REISBERG'S STAGES FOR EARLY DEMENTIA

This is also known as the **Global Deterioration Scale (GDS).** This is a tool used for determining the levels of cognitive function in a person with Alzheimer's disease or dementia. There are seven levels to this scale. Stages 1–3 identify the stages of predementia. Stages 4–7 identify the stages of dementia, with Stage 5 being the level that a person can no longer safely care for themselves independently.

| Stage | Symptoms |
| --- | --- |
| (1) No memory issues | No complaints of memory issues. No concerns noted by family, patient or during evaluations. |
| (2) Age-related memory decline | Forgetting names and forgetting where you place items or why you walked in to a room. Still able to complete work tasks, and safety is not a concern. |
| (3) Mild cognitive deficits | Earliest beginning signs that there may be deficits or issues. The patient may get confused in a new or unfamiliar location, have difficulty retaining new information such as a person's name or have difficulty meeting deadlines or completing tasks at work or putting valuable items in a "safe place" and not knowing where they were put. Patient begins to notice issues but is usually in denial and begins to show some signs and symptoms of anxiety. |
| (4) Moderate cognitive deficits/early dementia | Deficits are able to be identified by family and during evaluations. Difficulty recalling personal information, dates, and current events. Trouble with multistep commands and tasks and beginning difficulty with managing financing and medications. Patient becomes less engaged, less participatory in activity, and denies deficits, at times making jokes to distract from information that is difficult to recall. |
| (5) Moderate to severe cognitive deficits/ moderate dementia | Patient requires assistance at this point. Unable to remember specific details about their lives, mostly remembering major events. They become disoriented to time, have difficulty identifying names of family unless they are very close such as a spouse or child, and have difficulty making choices if there are more than two options. Driving becomes unsafe, there is difficulty in new environments, and safety deficits and impulsivity are common. |

| Stage | Symptoms |
|---|---|
| (6) Severe cognitive deficits/ moderately severe dementia | Often in this phase the spouse or children become the primary caregivers and are not recognized by the patient as a family member. Oftentimes, personalities change, frequent aggressiveness and difficult behaviors emerge, days and nights get confused, and you see the beginning of sundowners. Facts about their lives are difficult to recall. Word finding issues emerge. Consistent help is needed with ADLs including dressing, bathing, and toileting. Patients wander and get lost, and obsessive behaviors emerge such as constant sorting of items or cleaning the same thing repeatedly. Safety precautions are needed to avoid falls or the patient getting out of the home and wandering into the street or falling downstairs. |
| (7) Severe cognitive deficits/severe dementia | In this final stage, there is significant loss of verbal communications skills and ADLs. The patient is usually incontinent and may forget how to complete simple tasks such as feeding themselves or walking. Often, developmental reflexes that were integrated in the first years of life reemerge. Patients will need 24/7 supervision for safety. |

## ELISABETH KÜBLER-ROSS' STAGES OF GRIEF

There are five stages in **Kübler-Ross' theory**: denial, anger, bargaining, depression, and acceptance. These stages are the emotional response that humans have when they are faced with loss or are given a terminal diagnosis.

| Stage | Description |
|---|---|
| Denial | Patient is in shock. Can't believe this is happening. Believes there must be a mistake. How is this possible? |
| Anger | Why me? I am a good person? Why are they fine and I am not? Anger and frustration are aimed at family, caregivers, and medical staff. |
| Bargaining | Trying to make a deal to make the issue go away. If I pray hard or do a good deed, this will go away. If I could just make it to this event, then I will be okay. |
| Depression | Life as you know it is forever changed. Mourning for the loss of ability and unhappy about the need for assistance from friends and family. |
| Acceptance | Death is inevitable, getting affairs in order, finding a new reality different than before. |

## CAUSES FOR BALANCE ISSUES AND FALLS IN THE ELDERLY

Falls are the most frequent reason for hospitalization in the elderly population. Falls can be caused by environmental issues and balance issues. Environmental issues can include throw rugs, poor lighting, lack of grab bars, or furniture that scoots or moves unexpectedly. Balance issues can be caused by medications, vertigo or inner ear infections, vision issues such as glaucoma or macular degeneration, neuropathy in the lower extremities, cardiac issues such as high/low blood pressure, arthritis, neurological diseases, or cancer treatments. Common intervention areas are home safety assessments, nighttime toileting routines, lower extremity (LE) weakness concerns, cognitive deficits, decreased sensory awareness, and fear of falling because of previous falls and medication side effects.

## LEARNED HELPLESSNESS

**Learned helplessness** is when an elderly adult begins to feel and act helpless often due to sudden loss, injury, or diagnosis. He or she begins to relinquish control over things that previously held value, affecting motivation and self-esteem. The person begins to retreat and not participate in activities. This often occurs when the family begins to do everything for the older individual making all decisions for their family member and removing their autonomy and independence. Occupational therapists (OTs) can address this in their plan of care by creating task-oriented groups, cooking groups, leisure exploration tasks, education groups, ADLs, and current-event groups. Finding out what has meaning to the patient and teaching him how to advocate for himself can address the issue of learned helplessness and reintegrate the patient to finding meaning in his or her life again.

## AGING IN PLACE

**Aging in place** means that an elderly person will maintain independence and remain in their own home and community for as long as possible and live life doing the activities they desire as they age. Occupational therapists (OTs) can help by completing home evaluations to identify safety concerns such as removing obstacles or introducing adaptations or mobility aids. The American Occupational Therapy Association (AOTA) now has a Specialty Certification in Environmental Modifications.

### AREAS TO ADDRESS WHEN AGING IN PLACE

The following are areas to address when aging in place:

| Home modifications | Physical aspects of the home that are affected by balance, coordination, endurance, strength, and problem solving. Toilet and chair heights, grab bars, ramps. |
| --- | --- |
| Fall prevention | Home modifications that can reduce falls such as better lighting, removing tripping hazards such as throw rugs, and managing $O_2$ tubing. |
| Community mobility | Driving evaluations, bus schedules, family and friends providing transport. |
| Caregiver assistance | Working with the patient's family to identify and understand what the meaningful occupations are to the patient. If the patient thinks that cooking is a meaningful task, how does the family assist to make this a safe task if the person is unsupervised? |
| Cognitive screen | Using testing to determine cognitive deficits, driver safety, sequencing, and medication management. |
| Mental health | Environment modification to promote relaxation and stress-free activity. Organization, sensory input, and meditation. |
| Social skills | Assisting in engaging in social activities and events, education in technology. (Can they use a cell phone or work the TV remote?) |
| Wellness and disease management | Setting up a reasonable exercise program. (Do they have a schedule for taking medications, checking blood sugar, etc.?) |

## CARDIAC PROCEDURES

**Cardioversion** - This is when an electrical shock is delivered to the heart to convert an abnormal heart rhythm back to a normal sinus rhythm. This is done chemically through the use of medication or with an electric shock thorough special pads applied externally to the skin of the chest and back.

**Sternotomy** - An incision made during heart surgery through the sternum for access to the heart. The sternum is wired back together to heal. Patients will have sternal precautions for ~3 months postsurgery. These precautions include no lifting more than 5 lbs (a little more than a half-gallon of milk), no pushing, no pulling, and no reaching behind or overhead.

**Angioplasty** - A balloon catheter is inserted and inflated to expand the blood vessel and surrounding structure to increase blood flow. Oftentimes, a stent is inserted at the same time to keep the vessel open permanently. Otherwise, the balloon is deflated and removed.

**Cardiac ablation** - A procedure that removes or scars tissue from around the heart that is causing an abnormal heart rhythm. This can be done during open heart surgery or with a tube inserted in the groin and threaded to the heart where heat or cold is used to destroy the tissue.

**Cardiomyoplasty** - A procedure for end-stage heart failure in which skeletal muscle from another part of the body (usually the latissimus dorsi muscle) is placed around the heart and activated by a pacemaker to increase the heart's ability to pump.

**Stent** - A stent is a tube that is inserted into a vessel to assist in keeping it open in order to increase blood flow.

**Cardiac catheterization** - A procedure that is used to diagnose and treat cardiovascular conditions. A catheter is inserted into an artery in the groin or the neck and is threaded into the heart.

**Coronary artery bypass graft (CABG)** - A heart bypass graft in which veins are taken (usually from the leg) and are used to reroute and make new paths around blocked arteries to increase blood flow to the heart.

## IMPORTANT TERMS

**Diastolic**: The bottom number in a blood pressure reading. This number measures the force of the blood against the artery wall when the heart relaxes and the ventricles of the heart fill with blood. A normal reading is 80.

**Systolic**: The top number of the blood pressure reading. This number measures the force of the blood against the artery walls when the ventricles push the blood out of the heart. A normal reading is 120.

**Atrial fibrillation (AFib)**: The most common irregular heartbeat. Feels like a fluttering or a "hummingbird" in the chest. The electrical impulses cause the atria to misfire.

**Hypertension (HTN)**: This is high blood pressure. It can be from lifestyle and genetics, or it can be disease-/condition-related. When the heart is pumping blood with too much force, this causes a strain on the vessels pushing on them and expanding them. If this is a long-term condition and is not treated, it can lead to a stroke or heart attack.

**Hypotension**: This is low blood pressure, which is indicated by a systolic reading of less than 90 and a diastolic reading of less than 60. It can be caused by medications, stress, and pain.

**Syncope**: Loss of consciousness or fainting. The most common causes are low blood pressure, dehydration, or straining with a bowel movement.

**Diaphoresis**: Excessive sweating for no reason with no clear connection to the level of activity or the environment.

**Tachypnea**: Abnormal and rapid breathing of more than 20 breaths per minute.

**Bradycardia**: This is a slow heart rate, which can cause blood to not circulate fast enough throughout the body. This is fewer than 60 beats per minute.

## DERMATOMES AND MYOTOMES

**Myotomes** and **dermatome**s are part of the somatic nervous system, which is part of the bigger peripheral nervous system. Dermatomes are areas of the skin innervated by a spinal nerve causing sensory input. These spinal nerves take signals back to the central nervous system and report sensations: heat, body position, pain, etc. There are 8 cervical (C1 has no dermatome), 12 thoracic, 5 lumbar, 5 sacral, and 1 coccygeal dermatomes. A myotome is the muscle group that the spinal nerve innervates. It signals the muscles to contract. There is no myotome at S3. Myotomes can be tested with manual muscle testing. Dermatomes can be tested using a pinprick for pain and a cotton swab for pressure.

Cervical nerve roots and the dermatomes and myotomes that they control:

| Nerve Root | Dermatome | Myotome |
|---|---|---|
| C1 | None | Neck flexion/extension |
| C2 | Temple/forehead | Neck flexion/extension |
| C3 | Neck, cheek, temples, and mandible | Lateral neck flexion |
| C4 | Upper shoulder, upper scapula, and clavicle | Shoulder elevation |
| C5 | Deltoid and anterior arm to the base of thumb | Shoulder abduction |
| C6 | Anterior arm and radial aspect of the hand and index finger | Elbow flexion and wrist extension |
| C7 | Lateral arm and forearm and middle and ring fingers | Elbow extension, wrist flexion, and finger extension |
| C8 | Medial arm and forearm and middle, ring, and little fingers | Finger flexion |
| T1 | Medial forearm and base of the little finger | Finger abduction |
| T2 | Medial upper arm to the elbow; pectoral muscle region and midscapula | None |
| T3 | Upper thorax | None |
| T4 | Upper thorax | None |
| T5 | Upper thorax and costal margins | None |
| T6 | Upper thorax and costal margins | None |
| T7 | Costal margins | None |
| T8 | Abdomen and lumbar regions | None |
| T9 | Abdomen and lumbar regions | None |
| T10 | Abdomen and lumbar regions | None |
| T11 | Abdomen and lumbar regions | None |
| T12 | Abdomen and lumbar regions | None |
| L1 | Low back and anterior proximal thigh | Hip flexion |
| L2 | Low back and anterior middle knee | Hip flexion |
| L3 | Low back, upper buttocks, anterior thigh and knee, and medial lower leg | Knee extension |
| L4 | Medial buttocks, lateral thigh, medial leg, dorsum of the foot, and the big toe | Ankle dorsi flexion |
| L5 | Buttocks, posterior and lateral thigh, lateral leg, dorsum of the foot, medial sole of the foot, and the first, second, and third toes | Hip extension |
| S1 | Buttocks, thigh, and posterior leg | Hip extension, knee flexion, ankle plantar-flexion, ankle eversion |

| Nerve Root | Dermatome | Myotome |
|---|---|---|
| S2 | Buttocks, thigh, and posterior leg | Hip extension, knee flexion, ankle plantar-flexion |
| S3 | Groin and medial thigh to the knee | None |
| S4 | Perineum, genitals, and lower sacrum | Bladder and rectum |

## IMPACT TO FUNCTION FROM LEVELS OF INJURY IN THE SPINAL CORD

The levels of injury and the impact to function in the spinal cord are as follows:

- **C1–C4**: Paralysis of all four limbs, may not breathe independently, speaking is impacted, no bowel/bladder control, total assist for ADLs, may be able to use a Sip-N-Puff motorized wheelchair. Hoyer/mechanical lift for transfers. Needs 24/7 assist; there is a high risk for skin breakdown, wounds, and respiratory issues.
- **C5**: May have the ability to breathe independently and may be able to flex at the shoulder but with some paralysis in the wrist and hands. Will need moderate assist with ADLs; could likely use a wheelchair with a modified hand control.
- **C6**: Breathing is weak but uses the diaphragm. Paralysis in the hands and below the waist. May be able to use tenodesis movement to grasp items. No control over bowel and bladder but can likely transfer with adaptive devices such as a slide board. Can use motorized chair and possibly adaptive driving.
- **C7**: May have some elbow extension and finger flexion, but dexterity deficits exist. Normal shoulder movement and can attend to most ADL tasks independently. No control over bowel and bladder but can use devices independently for toileting. May use a manual wheelchair and drive adaptive vehicles.
- **C8**: Will have some hand movement, can grasp and release items without the use of tenodesis, but will have dexterity and fine motor skill deficits. Normal shoulder movement and can attend to most ADLs independently. No control over bowel and bladder but can use devices independently for toileting. May use a manual wheelchair and drive adaptive vehicles.
- **L1–L5**: This impacts the hips, thighs, genitals, and feet. Breathing and speech are not affected. Will likely be able to complete most ADLs independently; arm and hand function is normal. Can use a manual wheelchair, drive a modified car, and will have good balance in the torso. May use a slide board to transfer or none at all. Will use a standing frame in therapy. Will have some sexual dysfunction. Still no control of bowel or bladder but is generally independent with self-catheterizing and bowel regimens.
- **S1–S5**: Loss of function in the hips and legs; most of the impact is in the bladder, genitals, and bowels. Braces are often used here based on strength testing, and some patients will be able to walk with support based on the level and severity of the injury. Generally independent with self-catheterizing and bowel regimens for toileting. Will have some sexual dysfunction. Can drive a modified car. There is no impact on upper extremity (UE) use, speaking, or breathing. May use a slide board or nothing at all for transfers.

## IMPACT TO FUNCTION IN THE THORACIC SPINAL CORD

In most cases, injuries here result in paraplegia. Affects the lower chest and abdomen. Breathing and speech are not affected. Will likely be able to complete most ADLs independently; arm and hand function is normal. Can use a manual wheelchair and drive a modified car but will have balance issues in the torso. Can often use a slide board for transfers and will do well using a standing frame in therapy. Still no control of bowel or bladder but is generally independent with self-catheterization and bowel regiments.

## CRANIAL NERVES

The cranial nerves are 12 pairs of nerves that come from the brain and brainstem and control the senses, muscles, and internal organs. Cranial nerve names, functions and types are as follows:

| Nerve | What It Controls | Sensory/Motor/Both |
|---|---|---|
| I Olfactory | Smell | S |
| II Optic | Sight | S |
| III Oculomotor | Moves the eye up, down, left, right and diagonally; adjusts the pupil and lens of the eye | M |
| IV Trochlear | Moves the eye up, down, left, right, and diagonally | M |
| V Trigeminal | Largest of the cranial nerves; chewing, face sensation. | B |
| VI Abducens | Moves the eye up, down, left, right, and diagonally | M |
| VII Facial | Facial expression and anterior two-thirds of the tongue | B |
| VIII Vestibulocochlear | Sound | S |
| IX Glossopharyngeal | Swallowing, saliva, and taste | B |
| X Vagus | Control of the peripheral nervous system | B |
| XI Accessory | Swallowing and movement of the head and neck | M |
| XII Hypoglossal | Speech and swallowing; tongue muscles | M |

Mnemonic for nerve names: Oh, once one takes the anatomy final, very good vacations are heavenly.

Mnemonic for whether nerves are sensory/motor/both: Some say my mother bought my brother some bad beer, my, my.

## OCCUPATIONAL PROFILES

The **occupational profile** is the first step in the evaluation process. It is used to gather information about the patient's occupational history, activities of daily living (ADLs), routines, roles, what they value, and their goals. It is often created with a team approach, getting input from all medical and therapy team members as well as the patient and family. It is used to identify the problem areas of the patient to be addressed during therapy sessions and determine what is important to the patient in order to keep the treatments client centered. Areas of this assessment include the following:

- Why are they seeking therapy?
- What are they good at and what are some barriers?
- What is important to the patient?
- What are the patterns, routines, and habits of daily life?
- What are the physical areas that are supportive or considered barriers (such as being in the small space under the bed for reading but being scared of how dark it is once under the bed)?

- What are the social supports/barriers (the mom is a stay-at-home mom, but a new baby is pulling her attention away)?
- What are their customs and beliefs (no TV, church activities only, no sports)?
- Personal context: age, gender, school grade, family involvement.
- Temporal impact: developmental stage, when they are most productive (after lunch he is lethargic and needs a nap, more productive after breakfast, corrected age issues).
- Priorities and goals: Improvement in social skills, ADLs, mobility, cognition, etc.

## COGNITIVE REHABILITATION/DYNAMIC INTERACTIONAL APPROACH

The **cognitive rehabilitation/dynamic interactional approach** was created by Joan Toglia (cognitive rehabilitation), and as the theory was expanded, it became the dynamic interactional approach. In this theory, functional performance is restored in patients with cognitive dysfunction by focusing on orientation, attention, visual processing, motor planning, cognition, occupational behaviors, and effort. This is a commonly used reference for treatment with brain-injured patients. Treatment sessions focus on how components of daily life work together to ensure cognitive processing and that learning styles, life experience, effort, and specific aspects of our daily tasks affect cognition.

## DATA-DRIVEN DECISION-MAKING FRAMEWORK

The **data-driven decision-making framework** was created by an OT named Roseann C. Schaaf. It has a focus on the use of observation, testing, and intervention results to guide and measure outcomes in treatment planning. This theory has an eight-step process that shows how data are used to develop client-centered, replicable interventions to guide and measure treatment outcomes. The steps are as follows: (1) Identify participation challenges, (2) conduct the assessment, (3) generate a hypothesis, (4) develop goals, (5) identify outcome measures, (6) develop the intervention, (7) conduct the intervention, and (8) measure the outcome and monitor.

## TOP-DOWN/BOTTOM-UP APPROACH IN THERAPY

The **top-down** or **bottom-up** approach is a technique used by therapists in order to determine a course of treatment for their patients. In a top-down approach, treatment is compensatory. The therapist will try to maximize the skills and abilities that the patient continues to have. It is holistic in nature and considers the whole person and how to address functional performance considering all aspects of the person. The goal is to achieve as much function, mastery, or competency as possible and to offset the effects of the disability or impairment. In a bottom-up approach, treatment is more restorative, looking to identify the cause of the deficit and "fix" it. The goal is to restore function in the skills needed to complete the task and function fully in the desired occupation and address the root cause of the issue, but not necessarily to gain independence in the task. A top-down approach is at the level of the disability, whereas the bottom-up approach is at the level of the impairment.

## MOHO FRAME OF REFERENCE

**The Model of Human Occupation (MOHO) frame of reference** is based on a theory by Mary Reilly and later adapted by Gary Kielhofner and Janice Burke. It started as a model of practice and has evolved since the 1980s into one of the top frames of reference in use by therapists today. In Reilly's theory, the terms occupational role and occupational behavior are interchangeable. She believed that habit training and the roles on the work-play rest continuum were the greatest influence in life: student, employee, spouse, etc. Kielhofner looks at volition, habituation, and performance capacity in order to determine the motor, cognitive, and emotional skills needed to interact in the environment while taking into consideration life experiences. MOHO is client centered and holistic in nature because it looks at why humans are motivated to do the things they want to do, the patterns this creates in their lives, and how well they can complete these activities that they are motivated to complete.

## BEHAVIORAL FRAME OF REFERENCE

In the **behavioral frame of reference,** behavioral modification is used to shape and develop new behaviors. A patient's concerning behavior is identified to determine the baseline ability. A reinforcer and reinforcement schedule are created, and often a token economy is used and then phased out as the behaviors become permanent. The goal is to adapt and alter behaviors to increase occupational performance in the desired occupation. Examples of this frame of reference in practice are toileting schedules in children, social interactions in mental health patients, and self-regulation concerns.

## ACQUISITIONAL FRAME OF REFERENCE

The **acquisitional frame of reference** was created by Anne Mosey. It focuses on the patient learning a specific skill in order to elicit the most optimal performance and mastery of the skill in their personal environment. There are five main areas of focus in this frame of reference. Nurture is valued more than nature, the therapist accepts the patient unconditionally and without judgment, learning the skill brings competence in that skill, there is no one skill that is more important than another skill, and repetition and practice are the keys to mastery.

## BIOMECHANICAL FRAME OF REFERENCE

The **biomechanical frame of reference** is the oldest frame of reference used in rehabilitation, and no one knows for sure who created it. It focuses on the specific impairments that limit occupational performance in the patient. This is based on the idea that voluntary movement and control of the body come from muscle strength, joint capability and range, as well as strength and endurance. Therapeutic exercise is used to improve ROM, strength, and endurance, which will lead to improvement in functional abilities, and it is why this is a common frame of reference and one of the most easily used in physical disability settings.

## BRUNNSTROM MOVEMENT THERAPY FRAME OF REFERENCE

The **Brunnstrom movement therapy frame of reference** was created by a physical therapist named Signe Brunnström. The theory is based on the belief that when the central nervous system (CNS) is damaged, synergistic movements and reflexes in early childhood development will reemerge as part of the recovery process. Patients are taught to use and voluntarily control the motor patterns and reflexes as part of treatment so that normal patterns of movements can eventually be attained. This is opposite to Bobath's NDT approach, which inhibits abnormal patterns of movement.

## REHABILITATIVE FRAME OF REFERENCE

The **rehabilitative frame of reference** was created by Catherine Trombly Latham. The main goal of this frame of reference is adaptation to facilitate independence. Engagement in occupation requires an adaptive technique and compensatory strategies to the environment and possibly the occupation. This is most often used for patients who will likely have a lengthy recovery time or whose disability is considered permanent. The most common interventions for therapists using this theory are adaptive equipment and devices, energy conservation techniques, home modifications, and work simplification through task analysis.

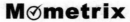

## DEVELOPMENTAL FRAME OF REFERENCE

The **developmental frame of reference** is based on normal human development. This theory was developed by an OT named Lela Llorens. It is used most often with gross motor and fine motor skill delays. Humans all develop at a different rate, but development is only considered "normal" and can move forward if each stage of development prior has been met. There are six adaptive skills in this theory: sensory skills, cognitive skills, dyadic interaction skills, group interaction skills, self-identity skills, and sexual identity skills. These areas need to be addressed in order for the patient to show a mastery of skills across all areas, and deficiencies in the development pattern and milestones must be addressed. Treatment sessions are based on assessing and addressing skills that are not mastered during developmental stages.

## SENSORY INTEGRATION FRAME OF REFERENCE

The **sensory integration frame of reference** was created by OT Jean Ayres. This frame of reference is based on how the brain receives sensory input from the environment and organizes it so that the body can respond with action. The focus on the senses, including auditory, vestibular, proprioceptive, tactile, and visual systems, provides information that contribute to a patient's learning and adaptive behaviors. There are four processing patterns of neurological thresholds and self-regulation that need to be addressed in this model. Is the patient sensory seeking, sensory avoiding, sensory sensitive, or do they have low registration? The goal of the therapist is to assist the patient in learning how to self-regulate input and modulate, discriminate, and integrate sensory information from the body and from the environment.

## NDT FRAME OF REFERENCE

The **neurodevelopmental treatment (NDT) frame of reference** was originally known as the Bobath approach and was developed by Berta and Karel Bobath. They believed that a therapist could have an impact on a client's functional movement by influencing the central nervous system through guided and specific handling techniques. At its core, it is used to analyze and treat posture and movement impairments based on kinesiology and biomechanics. Treatment sessions involve hands-on manipulation of posture and limbs in specific patterns to decrease muscle tone through the use of reflex inhibiting postures and techniques such as tapping and intermittent compression to provide proprioceptive and tactile stimulation.

## ROOD FRAME OF REFERENCE

The **Rood frame of reference** was created by OT Margaret Rood. This is a neurological treatment in which motor patterns are facilitated and normalized through sensory stimulation to specific sensory receptors. Treatment involves a developmental sequence designed by Rood that directs a patient's mobility using synergy patterns and controlled motion. Treatment can include manipulation and positioning of the body and limbs, joint compression, stimulating reflexes, and stretching muscles with and without resistance. Additionally, techniques using brushing, vibration, stroking, deep pressure, icing, and heat are used to achieve the greatest level of muscular response. In this theory, there are three major reactions that will occur in response to stimulation of specific receptors using the techniques listed above. (1) A homeostatic response will affect the autonomic nervous system by increasing or decreasing the patient's arousal levels. (2) A protective response is triggered, eliciting a protective or withdrawal response. (3) An adaptive response creates integration of multiple responses in the nervous system.

## ALLEN COGNITIVE DISABILITIES MODEL

**The Allen Cognitive Disabilities Model** was developed by an OT named Claudia K. Allen in the 1960s. This model helps us identify a person's functional cognition at every stage of dementia so

34

that we can focus on current abilities instead of what a person can no longer do. There are 0–6 Allen cognitive levels (ACLs) in this model that help identify remaining abilities. There are now tools and screens used to support this model including the Allen Cognitive Level Screen (ACLS-5) and the Allen Diagnostic Module.

| Level | Description |
|---|---|
| ACL 0: Coma | Generalized reflexive actions |
| ACL 1: Awareness | Level of arousal observed as a specific response to an external stimulus. |
| ACL 2: Gross body movements | The awareness to own proprioceptive cues of body position in space and against gravity. |
| ACL 3: Manual actions | The manual actions in response to tactile cueing. |
| ACL 4: Familiar activity | Being aware of tangible cues and can understand cause and effect. |
| ACL 5: Learning new activity | Understanding deductive reasoning and learning new tasks through trial and error. |
| ACL 6: Planning new activity | No impairment of cognitive deficits is noted. Can plan and prepare for activity, learn new tasks, and safety concerns are anticipated and avoided. |

## CANADIAN MODEL OF OCCUPATIONAL PERFORMANCE

The **Canadian model of occupational performance** was created by the Canadian Association of Occupational Therapists in the 1980s. It is a client-centered therapy focused on occupational performance, and it has three core areas: the person, environment and occupation. The person is at the center of this model and represents how spirituality is influenced by affective, physical, and cognitive abilities at the core of a person's being and motivation. The middle ring is occupation, and it includes the three domains of self-care, productivity, and leisure. The outer ring is environment, and it shows the influence of the physical, social, cultural, and institutional impact on the patient. As a whole, the interactions between the person, environment, and occupation are what make the occupational performance. From this theory, the **Canadian Occupational Performance Measure (COPM)** was created. It is an evidence-based outcome measure designed to determine a patent's self-perception of occupational performance in everyday living.

## EHP MODEL

The **ecology of human performance (EHP)** model was created by OT Winnie Dunn. It identifies that human performance is affected by the context in which the performance takes place. What this means is that the context and environment where tasks are learned can provide important cues and reinforcement in occupational tasks. The four core pieces of this theory are person, task, context, and performance. A person is a unique being that has experiences, skills, and abilities and is embedded in context and therefore can't be understood out of the context. The tasks are activities that need to be completed in order to obtain a goal. Context can be cultural, physical, temporal, and social in nature. Context is fluid and is always changing based on personal experience. People perform tasks within a context using their skills and abilities based on their abilities, skills, and interests. Performance is based on past experiences and resources.

## LPM MODEL

The **lifestyle performance model (LPM)** was created by OT Gail Fidler. This is a theory for understanding a person's occupational performance within the context of his own life experience. This is one of the most common frameworks in occupational therapy because it was the first to identify that quality of life is key to measuring human performance. This framework introduced the

35

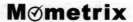

term **lifestyle performance**, which is a holistic way of looking at occupational performance. Lifestyle performance is the ability to engage in all activities in daily life without just focusing on self-care tasks. A person's total activity range is considered within the context of that person's world.

## PERSON-ENVIRONMENT-OCCUPATION-PERFORMANCE MODEL

The **Person-Environment-Occupation-Performance** model was created by OTs Gary Christiansen and Carolyn Baum. It uses the interaction among the person, abilities, environment, and occupational influences to determine treatment and performance outcomes. This is a unique patient-centered and holistic frame of reference because it considers the physical, emotional, and social factors that can influence someone's occupational performance. It is a top-down rather than bottom-up model. It can be used as an assessment and as an intervention model. The overlapping area of the three domains shapes occupational performance and shows the interaction between the person, environment, and occupation.

# Analysis and Interpretation

## EBP

**Evidence-based practice (EBP)** is how clinical expertise is integrated with clinical evidence from systematic research. More simply put, it is based on a combination of research results, clinical expertise, and the client's preferences, beliefs, and values. Therapists are under increasing pressure to justify the services they provide because of reimbursement issues, services provided within the scope of practice, and staffing ratios: EBP is how this is done. The EBP process has six steps: (1) formulating the clinical question, (2) searching for the best available evidence, (3) critically analyzing evidence for its validity and usefulness, (4) integrating the appraisal with personal clinical expertise and clients' preferences, (5) evaluating performance or outcomes of actions, and (6) disseminating and communicating knowledge so that the entire profession benefits.

## Physical and Psychosocial Determinants of Occupation

When an OT is looking at patients' needs using the **physical determinants of occupation**, the overall musculoskeletal system is taken into consideration. Strength, ROM, and endurance are addressed in order to best meet the patient's needs. The ability to evaluate stamina and physical demands to complete occupational performance and task is key. As a therapist, your sessions would likely include strengthening, endurance, activity tolerance, balance, pacing, coordination, and overall exercises in order to address functional mobility and ADLs. When a therapist is looking at patients' needs using the **psychosocial determinants of occupation**, the patient's thoughts, feelings, and emotions that could be impacting functional performance are taken into consideration. The context of people's lives has a large impact on their overall health and well-being. People see things and react through the lens of their own experiences. Personal circumstances and environment make a difference in the outcome of the treatment plan that the therapist creates for the patient. Treatment would likely include cognitive evaluation, stress relievers, coping mechanisms, problem solving, relaxation techniques, projective techniques, and basic skills training in order to address functional mobility, cognition, and ADLs.

## Therapeutic Use of Self

Therapeutic use of self is when a therapist uses his personality and personal experiences and skills to build rapport with his patient. This builds a relationship with the patient in which the patient can feel comfortable sharing and builds trust so that they can focus on their treatment. In some ways, therapists become chameleons by adapting to fit the needs of a client. The therapist needs to be aware of visual and verbal cues and how much personal information he or she is willing to share so as to not cross professional boundaries. During the evaluation, the therapist needs to collect as much insight on a patient as possible. The patient's communication style alone can set the groundwork for successful participation and rapport. Notice if the patient speaks loudly or quietly; what is the tone; how much personal space does the patient require; and what is the patient's use of humor, short words, complex wording, slang, bluntness, and sarcasm. Can you meet their level of communication in order to make the patient comfortable? Are they comfortable being told how to complete an activity seeing the therapist as the expert, or do they need to feel more give and take by having more of a say in their treatment? Determine how much personal experience you are willing to share without making yourself or the patient uncomfortable. Did you go through cancer treatment and feel that sharing your experience will help build comradery? Are you a parent? Have you traveled to their home state or city? Have you broken your leg before? The goal is to make your patient as comfortable as possible to get the best results from therapy without lying and also not making it all about you.

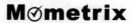

## COGNITIVE NEUROLOGICAL DETERMINANTS OF OCCUPATION

When a therapist is looking at patients' needs using the **cognitive neurological determinants of occupation**, he or she looks at how the central nervous system affects and impacts occupational performance. More specifically, we focus on memory, motor planning, attention to task, balance, coordination, sensory perception, executive functioning, and neuroplasticity. Assessments during evaluation would include a combination of interview, observation, as well as cognitive testing and balance and coordination testing. Sessions would likely include home modifications, adaptive equipment training, ADL training and functional adaptation, balance and fall prevention, memory aids, sensory retraining, and pain management.

## SOCIAL, CULTURAL, AND ECONOMIC DETERMINANTS OF OCCUPATION

Looking at the **social, cultural, and economic determinants of occupation**, a therapist needs to be aware of how the roles, habits, and beliefs of the patient impact occupation. The greatest impact on occupation is often not disability but the influence of income levels and poverty, employment and occupation, education, housing, culture, and ethnicity. Treatment needs to consider the demands and expectations of occupational performance. Culturally, is it reasonable to expect your male patient to cook his own meals and do laundry to return home, or is it expected that his children will do this for him? Does the patient live in a house and have funds available to make major environmental changes for ease in mobility and ADLs, or does she live in a small apartment where she can't make structural changes to the home? These roles will impact what is reasonable and attainable in goal setting. Treatment will always be influenced by these factors, so the expectations of the patient and family need to be addressed at the evaluation.

## FUNCTIONAL MOBILITY VS. GAIT TRAINING

**Functional mobility** is a person's ability to move around in his or her environment. This can include ambulation with and without a device, transferring from surface to surface (chair to commode), and bed mobility. **Gait training** involves analyzing the pattern of how a person walks with a detailed focus on step length, stride length, speed, trunk rotation, and arm swing. This is within the physical therapy scope of practice. Functional mobility is within the scope of practice of occupational therapy, whereas gait training is not. External reviewers will deny gait training services when provided by an OT. Functional mobility in occupational therapy will teach a patient how to safely ambulate in their environment during a functional task for increased independence and safety during ADL activity. It is well within the scope of OT practice to address areas that impact functional performance and safety, regardless of mobility level.

## SENSORY PROFILE

The **sensory profile** is a norm-referenced, standardized questionnaire assessment designed by OT Winnie Dunn to address sensory processing patterns of children and adults. There are six versions of this test based on the age of the patient. They are the infant sensory profile with a caregiver questionnaire for babies from birth–6 months, toddler sensory profile 2 with a caregiver questionnaire for toddlers ages 7–35 months, child sensory profile with a caregiver questionnaire for children ages 3–14 years, short sensory profile with a caregiver questionnaire for children ages 3–14 years, school companion sensory profile with a teacher questionnaire for students ages 3–14 years old, and the adolescent/adult sensory profile with a questionnaire to address ages 11 and older. Eight areas of sensory input are examined on all the tests, including auditory, visual, activity level, taste/smell, body position, movement, touch, and emotional/social. Items are given a score based on the caregiver's indication of how often the behavior is seen: almost always, frequently, occasionally, seldom, or almost never. These scores get added up, and the number indicates if the patient falls into a typical performance pattern, probable difference, or definite difference in correlation to his peer group. Often, the results of this exam will lead to the creation of a sensory diet for the patient to address attention, arousal, and adaptive responses for integration in daily life.

## SENSORY DIET

A **sensory diet** is an activity plan that provides the sensory input that a person needs to stay focused and organized throughout the day. These plans are generally created based on the results of the sensory profile. Tasks and activities in the "diet" can include activities that encourage sensations and situations that are challenging, increasing alertness, regulating emotions, decreasing unwanted sensory seeking or avoiding behaviors, and working through transitions during work and play. This is a tool most often used with children on the autism spectrum or with sensory processing issues, but it is also being used working with adults dealing with the symptoms and issues of dementia and Alzheimer's disease, including adverse behaviors. Examples of this can be heavy work for proprioception such as lifting, pushing, and pulling items; vestibular input such as spinning and swinging; auditory input such as noise-canceling headphones or music can be played; and olfactory activities such as "scent breaks" in which cotton balls saturated in scents such as orange or peppermint or vanilla can be inhaled for a calming effect. These activities can be done throughout the day and integrated into work or play activities.

## PLANES OF MOTION USED WHEN TESTING ROM IN A PATIENT

There are three different planes of motion: **sagittal, frontal, and transverse.** In each of these planes, several different movements occur at the joints. The frontal plane passes through the body from left to right, dividing the body into anterior and posterior. The transverse plane passes through the body in a line parallel to the floor, dividing the body into top and bottom. The sagittal plane passes through the body from front to back, dividing the body into left and right.

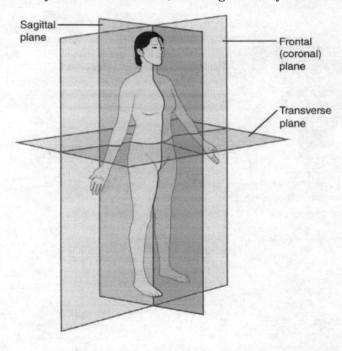

## MOVEMENT IN THE SAGITTAL PLANE OF MOTION

The sagittal plane passes through the body from front to back, dividing the body into left and right sides.

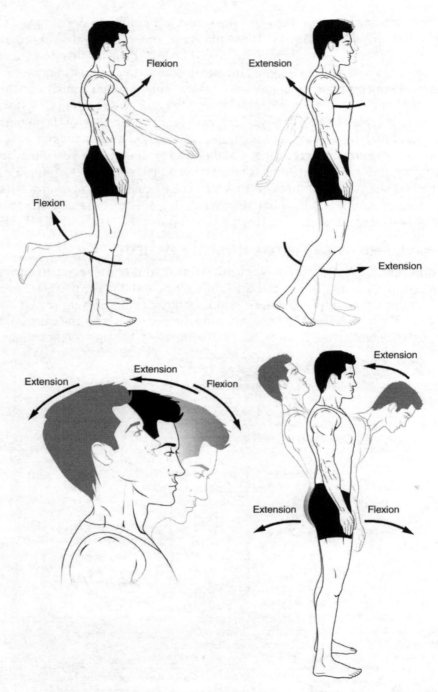

| Flexion | Decrease the angle between two body parts (bending the elbow) |
| Extension | Increasing the angle between two body parts (straightening the elbow) |
| Dorsiflexion | Ankle flexion (moving the toes toward the shin) |
| Plantar flexion | Ankle extension (moving the toes toward the ground/pointing the toes) |

40

### MOVEMENT IN THE FRONTAL PLANE OF MOTION

The frontal plane passes through the body from left to right, dividing the body into anterior and posterior.

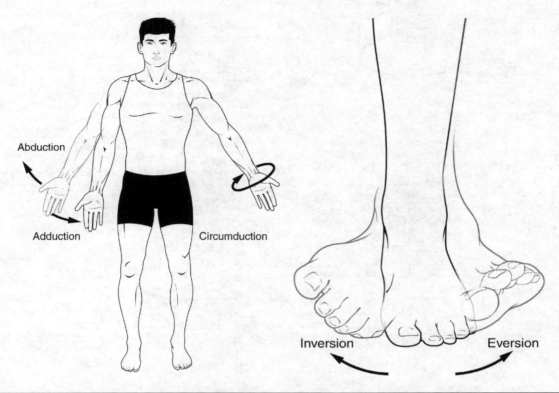

| Adduction | Movement toward the midline/to the body (bringing your arm to your body). |
| Abduction | Moving away from the midline Think of someone being abducted or taken away (moving your arm away from the body). |
| Elevation | Scapula movement, superior movement (shoulder shrug). |
| Depression | Scapula movement, inferior movement (shoulder shrug). |
| Inversion | Lifting the medial border of your foot. You bring the sole of the foot to face inward. |
| Eversion | Lifting the lateral border of your foot. You bring the sole of the foot to face outward. |

## MOVEMENT IN THE TRANSVERSE PLANE OF MOTION

The transverse plane passes through the body in a line parallel to the floor, dividing the body into top and bottom.

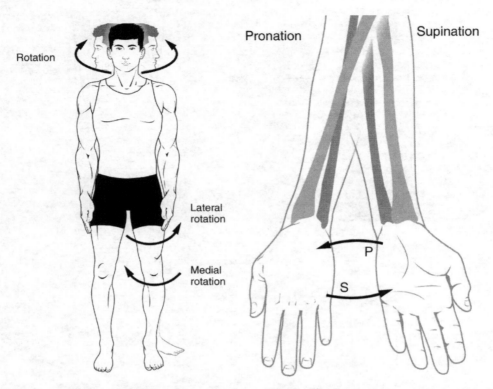

| Pronation | Rotating the hand and wrist medially from the bone. If laying on your back, the hand would have the palm to the floor. |
| Supination | Rotating the hand and wrist laterally from the bone. If laying on your back, the palm and wrist would be facing toward the ceiling. |
| Horizontal adduction | The angle between two joints decreases on the horizontal plane. |
| Horizontal abduction | The angle between two joints increases on the horizontal plane. |
| Rotation | Pivoting or twisting on the axis (turning the head left or right). |

## ASSESSING ROM

**Range of motion (ROM)** is the measurement of movement around a specific joint or body part. This is assessed by a therapist using observation, palpation, and the use of a tool called a goniometer. ROM can be assessed actively (AROM) or passively (PROM). AROM is when the patient actively contracts the muscles to move through ROM independently. PROM is when the therapist moves the patient through the full ROM without assistance from the patient. The goal is to look for the presence of pain during the movement and the actual range of movement that we measure in degrees. When ROM is limited, it can affect the patient's functioning and cause pain. We look at end feel during this process. **End feel** is when the movement is stopped or resisted when passively moving the joint through the end of its ROM reaching its limit. End feel can be soft, firm, or hard. **Soft end feel** is seen in knee and elbow flexion where there is soft-tissue approximation. **Firm end feel** is when there is a normal stretch and is seen in finger extension and arm pronation. **Hard end feel** is bone to bone and is seen in elbow extension.

## ROM PARAMETERS OF THE UE AND NECK

The following are the normal ROM parameters for each joint in the UE and neck:

| Movement | ROM | End Feel |
|---|---|---|
| Neck rotation | 0°–80° | Firm end feel |
| Neck flexion | 0°–50° | Firm end feel |
| Neck extension | 0°–60° | Firm end feel |
| Shoulder flexion | 0°–150° | Firm end feel |
| Shoulder extension | 0°–50° | Firm end feel |
| Shoulder abduction | 0°–150° | Firm end feel |
| Shoulder adduction | 0°–30° | Firm end feel |
| Elbow flexion | 0°–150° | Soft end feel |
| Elbow extension | 0° | Hard end feel |
| Forearm supination | 0°–80° | Firm end feel |
| Forearm pronation | 0°–80° | Hard/Firm end feel |
| Wrist flexion | 0°–60° | Firm end feel |
| Wrist extension | 0°–60° | Firm end feel |
| Wrist radial deviation | 0°–20° | Hard/Firm end feel |
| Wrist ulnar deviation | 0°–30° | Firm end feel |

## ROM PARAMETERS OF THE LEs, ANKLE, AND BACK

The following are the normal ROM parameters for each joint in the lower extremities (LEs), ankle, and back:

| Movement | ROM | End Feel |
|---|---|---|
| Back extension | 0°–25° | Firm end feel |
| Back flexion | 0°–90° | Firm end feel |
| Back lateral flexion | 0°–25° | Firm end feel |
| Hip extension | 0°–30° | Firm end feel |
| Hip flexion | 0°–100° | Soft end feel |
| Hip abduction | 0°–40° | Firm end feel |
| Hip adduction | 0°–20° | Firm end feel |
| Knee flexion | 0°–150° | Soft end feel |
| Ankle inversion | 0°–30° | Hard end feel |
| Ankle eversion | 0°–20° | Hard end feel |
| Ankle plantarflexion | 0°–40° | Hard/Firm end feel |
| Ankle dorsiflexion | 0°–20° | Firm end feel |

## ROM PARAMETERS OF THE HAND

The following are the normal ROM parameters for each joint in the hand:

| Joint | ROM |
|---|---|
| Metacarpophalangeal (MCP) abduction | 0°–25° |
| MCP adduction | 20°–0° |
| MCP flexion | 0°–90° |
| MCP extension | 0°–30° |
| Proximal interphalangeal (PIP) flexion | 0°–120° |
| PIP extension | 120°–0° |
| Distal interphalangeal (DIP) flexion | 0°–80° |

43

| Joint | ROM |
|---|---|
| DIP extension | 80°–0° |
| MCP joint of the thumb abduction | 0°–50° |
| MCP joint of the thumb adduction | 40°–0° |
| MCP joint of the thumb flexion | 0°–70° |
| MCP joint of the thumb extension | 60°–0° |
| Interphalangeal (IP) joint of the thumb flexion | 0°–90° |
| IP joint of the thumb extension | 90°–0° |

## COMPLETING STRENGTH TESTING IN A THERAPY EVALUATION

**Manual muscle testing (MMT)** and the use of a dynamometer (for pinch and grip) are the most common methods to measure strength in a therapy evaluation. We do this to evaluate the strength of a muscle or muscle group to determine the ability to move against gravity and with resistance in the full and available ROM. Muscles can be graded into six categories: zero (0), trace (1), poor (2), fair (3), good (4), and normal (5). In the zero category, no muscle contraction can be felt. In the trace category, the muscle contraction can be palpated but you may not see active movement. In the poor category, movement is available but only with gravity eliminated. In the fair, normal, and good categories, full ROM is seen against gravity. Further strength is identified in the good and normal categories because the muscle can sustain movement and hold its position with resistance in addition to moving against gravity. Each category can be adjusted by using a (+) or (−) system, and it is designated in the chart.

| Description | Abv. | Number | Gravity | ROM | Resistance |
|---|---|---|---|---|---|
| Normal | N | 5 | Against | Full | Maximum |
| Good | G | 4 | Against | Full | Moderate |
| Good Minus | G- | 4- | Against | Full | Less than Mod. |
| Fair Plus | F+ | 3+ | Against | Full | Minimal with breaks |
| Fair | F | 3 | Against | Full | None |
| Fair Minus | F- | 3- | Against | >50% | None |
| Poor Plus | P+ | 2+ | Against | <50% | None |
| Poor Plus | P+ | 2+ | Eliminated | Full | Minimal with breaks |
| Poor | P | 2 | Eliminated | Full | None |
| Poor Minus | P- | 2- | Eliminated | <Full | None |
| Trace | T | 1 | | | |
| Zero | 0 | 0 | | | |

## PROCESS OF GRIP AND PINCH STRENGTH TESTING

**Grip and pinch strength testing** is an important part of a therapy evaluation in an outpatient setting. It helps to establish a baseline for treatment, grade tasks, determine what tasks a patient can or cannot functionally complete, monitors progress, and helps set realistic and attainable goals for therapy. These tests are often used when a patient is referred to therapy after and upper extremity (UE) or hand surgery, tendon or nerve damage, stroke, cerebral palsy (CP), multiple sclerosis (MS), Parkinson's, or osteoarthritis (OA). Grip strength is measured using a hand dynamometer. The patient is to sit in a low-back chair with forearms on the arms of the chair and feet flat on the floor. The wrists should be just over the end of the chair's arm, thumbs facing upward. Patients will position their thumb around one side and their fingers around the other side of the handle and squeeze. When the needle stops rising, read the measurement from the dial and record the result. The outside dial usually registers in kilograms and the inner dial in pounds. A pinch test is administered from a pinch gauge, and it measures the tip pinch (thumb tip to index

44

fingertip), key pinch/lateral pinch (thumb pad to lateral aspect of the middle phalanx of index finger), and palmar pinch/three-jaw chuck pinch (thumb pad to the pads of the index and middle fingers).

## BRUININKS-OSERETSKY TESTS OF MOTOR PROFICIENCY (BOT-2)

The **Bruininks-Oseretsky Tests of Motor Proficiency (BOT-2)** is a standardized test used to evaluate fine and gross motor skills, and it can be used with typically developing children and children with developmental disabilities between the ages of 4 and 21. This test has a complete form and a short form, and it has four sections with eight subtests that include fine manual control, manual coordination, body coordination, and strength and agility. The short form has 14 items selected from the subtests of the complete form, and it is most often used to screen for further evaluation. The complete form takes 40–60 minutes to administer, and the short form takes 15–20 minutes.

## FUNCTIONAL REACH TEST

The **functional reach test** is a criterion-referenced standardized test. The purpose is to assess forward functional reach in a fixed position. The test is completed five times with two practices and three actual tests. A yardstick is affixed to a wall, and the patient's arm is extended to 90° shoulder level. The patient is asked to "reach as far as you can forward without taking a step," and the location of the third metacarpal is recorded. Typical functional reach is 10 inches or greater. Scores of less than 7 inches of reach indicate limited functional balance, and scores of less than 6 inches of reach indicate a high fall risk.

## TUG TEST

The **timed "up and go" (TUG) test** assesses fall risk in adults by looking at how long it takes to complete standing from a seated position, walking, turning, and sitting down. Standardized cutoff scores to predict risk of falling have not been established in research, and there are no formal normal values. However, older adults who take longer than 13.5 seconds to complete the TUG test have a high risk for falling, with **19 seconds** or more associated with increased risk of having multiple falls. The therapist times the patient when they stand up from a chair, walk 10 feet, turn around, walk back, and sit down with or without the use of device. The test is used in multiple settings, and it requires only a chair and a stopwatch to complete.

## FIST AND 30-SECOND SIT-TO-STAND ASSESSMENT

The **Function in Sitting Test (FIST)** is a criterion-referenced standardized test created to assess seated bedside balance and stability after stroke or brain injury. It has 14 items, and it is scored from 0 to 4, with the numbers indicating (0) dependent, (1) needs assistance, (2) UE support, (3) verbal cues/increased time, and (4) independent. The patient sits on the edge of the bed with hands in the lap and with the feet supported. The patient is given sternal nudges, asked to scoot, pick up an item from the floor, sit with eyes closed, lift feet from the floor, reach for items, and shake head yes/no while maintaining balance. The **30-second chair test** evaluates leg strength and endurance. The patient is seated in a chair with a straight back without armrests with a seat 17 inches high and asked to complete as many sit-to-stands as he can without using his arms in a 30-second time frame. Scores are based on age for both men and women, and a below-average score indicates a risk for falls.

## SEMMES-WEINSTEIN MONOFILAMENT TEST

The Semmes-Weinstein monofilament test is a sensory assessment that is used to test for nerve compression syndromes, peripheral neuropathy, thermal injuries, and postoperative nerve repair deficits in the extremities. The tool has multiple monofilaments in different sizes. Green is equivalent to normal sensation, blue is equivalent to a diminished light touch sensation, purple is equivalent to diminished protective sensation, red is equivalent to loss of protective sensation, and the red striped lines mean that sensation is untestable in that region. Testing begins with having the patient rest the extremity being tested on a table and having them close their eyes and say "yes" when they feel something. Each test has a guide of where to test on the patient and the order of testing. Generally, the testing will move from digit one to digit five, distally to proximally, anteriorly to posteriorly, and then the volar palm and dorsal hand are tested, and the anterior then posterior forearm for the UE. The therapist will press the filament at a 90° angle against the skin until it bows and will keep it in place for 1.5 seconds.

## COORDINATION

**Coordination** is the ability to complete smooth, accurate, and controlled motor responses on demand. Coordination encompasses gross motor skills, fine motor skills, and hand-eye coordination skills. This can be the UE moving smoothly to create gross or fine dexterity movement for handwriting, or it can be how the body moves through space organized and not tripping or bumping into objects in the environment. Bilateral coordination is the ability to use both sides of the body together in a coordinated way. This is seen in tying shoes, using a knife and fork, and running. To test UE coordination, therapists will often have the patient try to button and unbutton an item or use the finger-to-nose test. In this test, the patient sits across from the therapist and takes the tip of his index finger to the tip of his nose and then moves his finger to the therapist's finger that is held in front of the patient. In the LE, a therapist would use a heel-to-shin test or have the patient walk along a straight line. In the heel-to-shin test, the patient will raise one leg and with their heel touch their opposite knee and drag the heel along the shin toward the ankle and then slowly back up to the knee.

## PROPRIOCEPTION

**Proprioception** is how we identify our body position in space. The sensory receptors in our skin, joints, and muscles help provide information for motor movement and postural control. When a patient has deficits in proprioception, they will like be labeled as "clumsy" or they will be at a high risk for falling. There are no standardized tests for proprioception, but there are two ways that therapists can test it. The therapist can stand behind the patient so they can't see you and what you are doing. The patient will then be requested to close their eyes, and the therapist will position one UE (including the hand, wrist, and fingers) in a position and have the patient attempt to copy the position with the opposite limb. The other testing option is to have the patient close his eyes and the therapist will move his limb into a flexed or extended position and back into neutral. The patient will then be asked to identify if the limb was flexed or extended after the movement has ended. Proprioception is documented in the evaluation as either impaired or intact.

## BEERY-VMI

The **Beery-Buktenica Developmental Test of Motor Integration (Beery-VMI)** is an assessment for ages 2 and up. The short form is geared for ages 2–7. It is a norm-referenced, standardized assessment used to assess deficits in visual perception, fine motor skills, and hand-eye coordination. It focuses on the patient's ability to integrate visual and motor skills, but it is also a top assessment to be used as an outcome measure to test improvements in visual–motor integration skills after handwriting interventions during treatments. The core of the test is copying 30 geometric forms with 2 subtests designed to look at visual abilities without the fine motor component and then fine motor skills without the use of visual perceptual skills. The test takes 10–15 minutes to complete.

## DTVP-2

The **Developmental Test of Visual Perception (DTVP-2)** is a standardized test with high reliability and validity used to test visual perception and visual-motor integration skills. It is used with children ages 4–10. The test takes 45 minutes to administer. There are 8 subtests that include hand-eye coordination, proprioception, copying, figure ground, spatial relationships, visual closure, visual motor speed, and form constancy. The test has been normed through age 75, and it has also been a helpful tool with TBI patients, right-hemisphere stroke patients, and patients with dementia.

## MVPT-4

The **Motor-Free Visual Perception Test (MVPT-4)** is a standardized test of visual perception. It can be used for ages 4–70. It tests the areas of visual discrimination, spatial relationship, visual memory, figure-ground, and visual closure. There are 36 cards with a 2D figure on them and choices from a to d to choose the item that most closely matches the example. The test takes 10–15 minutes to administer. It is most often used in the pediatric setting and as an indicator for driver recertification after stroke or head injury.

### TWO-POINT DISCRIMINATION TEST AND THE NINE-HOLE PEG TEST

The two-point discrimination test is a standardized test used to assess if the patient is able to identify two close points on a small area of skin, and it determines how fine the ability to discriminate this is after injury or surgery. It is most commonly used after hand surgery, grafts, nerve repairs, and tissue transfer for desensitization and to determine the level of impairment. The therapist requests that the patient closes his eyes and then states: "I will touch you with either one or two points, and tell me if you feel one or two points when you feel the touch." The nine-hole peg test is a standardized test used to measure finger dexterity. It is used after hand surgery to improve and monitor dexterity, and it is also used to assess patients with stroke, brain injury, Parkinson's disease, and multiple sclerosis (MS). The test is given four times: twice with the dominant hand and twice with the nondominant hand. The patient is timed picking up nine pegs, one at a time as quickly as possible, and putting them in the nine holes on the board. Once they are placed in the holes, he removes them again as quickly as possible one at a time, replacing them into the container at the other end of the peg board. The total time to complete the task is recorded.

### BATTELLE DEVELOPMENTAL INVENTORY

The **Battelle Developmental Inventory** is an assessment for infants and children through age 7. It is a flexible, semi-structured assessment that uses observation of the child and interviews with parents and caregivers. The test has 5 global developmental areas and 13 categories to evaluate strengths and deficits in personal-social, adaptive, motor, communication, and cognitive skill sets. This test is aligned with the federal requirements for the Office of Special Education Programs and the Head Start Program, and it indicates readiness for school or a need for special education services. The test can be completed in 60–90 minutes.

## FIM

The **Functional Independence Measure (FIM)** is a standardized test that is used in order to address the physical, psychological, and social functioning of a patient. There are 18 categories in this test broken into motor and cognition sections, and it takes approximately 60 minutes to administer. It is used primarily in skilled nursing facilities (SNFs) or in an acute rehabilitation setting in order to assess a patient's level of disability during the evaluation process and to monitor changes in the patient's status in response to treatment interventions. Each item on the FIM is scored on a scale from 1 to 7. The higher the score, the more independent the patient is in performing the task. A score of 1 is total assistance with a helper. A score of 2 is maximal assistance

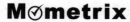

with helper. A score of 3 is moderate assistance with a helper. A score of 4 is minimal assistance with helper. A score of 5 is supervision or setup with a helper. A score of 6 is modified independence with no helper. A score of 7 is complete independence with no helper.

## CATEGORIES OF THE FIM AND THE AREAS OF SCORING FOR THE ADL ITEMS

There are 18 items on the functional independence measure (FIM) organized into 2 categories: motor and cognitive. The motor category is comprised of eating, grooming, bathing, upper body dressing, lower body dressing, toileting, bladder management, bowel management, transfers (bed/chair/wheelchair), transfers (toilet), transfers (bath/shower), ambulation (walking/wheelchair), and stairs. The cognitive category is comprised of comprehension, expression, social interactions, problem solving, and memory. There are six activities of daily living (ADL) areas that cover the following tasks:

| Category | Categories of Scoring |
|---|---|
| Feeding | Picking up a utensil, using suitable utensils, scooping food onto a utensil, bringing food to the mouth, drinking from a cup or glass, chewing and swallowing, managing a variety of food consistencies. |
| Grooming | Oral care, hair grooming (combing or brushing), washing hands, washing the face, shaving the face or applying make-up. |
| Bathing | Left arm, chest, right arm, abdomen, front perineal area, back perineal area (buttocks), left upper leg, right upper leg, left lower leg including the foot, right lower leg including the foot. |
| Upper body dressing | Shirt, right arm, left arm, overhead, arranging in the back, fasteners; bra, right arm, left arm, overhead, arranging in the back, fasteners; and sweater/jacket, right arm, left arm, overhead, arranging in the back, fasteners. |
| Lower body dressing | Pants, right leg, left leg, arranging over hips, fasteners; socks, right foot, left foot; shoes, right foot, left foot, fastener; underwear/brief, right leg, left leg, arranging over hips; and compression stockings, right foot, left foot. |
| Toileting | Transfer, clothing management, hygiene. |

## KATZ INDEX OF INDEPENDENCE IN ACTIVITIES OF DAILY LIVING

The **Katz Index of Independence in Activities of Daily Living** is used to assess functional status and the ability to perform ADLs independently. The test is not standardized, and there is no formal reliability or validity research, but it is a common test used in multiple settings. The index ranks performance in six areas: bathing, dressing, toileting, transferring, continence, and feeding. Patients are given a score of yes/no for independence in each area. A high score of 6 points is possible. A score of 6 identifies independence, a score of 3–5 is partially dependent or moderate assistance needed, and a score of 2 or less identifies dependence in the activity and severe functional impairment.

## PDMS-2

The **Peabody Developmental Motor Scales (PDMS-2)** is a standardized and norm-referenced test used to assess gross and fine motor skills in children from birth to age 5. It takes 60 minutes to complete the entire test, but each component can be administered individually in 20–30 minutes. There are six areas of the test.

| Test Area | What the Area Tests |
|---|---|
| Reflexes | Addresses how the child automatically reacts to environmental events. This component is only given to children ages 2 weeks through 11 months because most reflexes are integrated after this age. |

48

| Test Area | What the Area Tests |
|---|---|
| Stationary | Looks at the control of the body within the child's center of gravity and his ability to retain equilibrium. |
| Locomotion | Looks at the child's mobility and how they move from one place to another. This can be crawling, walking, running, hopping, and/or jumping. |
| Object manipulation | Addresses the child's ability to catch and throw items. This component is only given to children ages 1 and older. |
| Grasping | This looks at the child's ability to use his hands. It starts with basic activity such as holding an object, and it progresses to manipulating in both hands and completing buttons and fasteners. |
| Visual-motor integration | Addresses a child's hand-eye coordination and visual perceptual skills. This component moves from basic reaching, grasping, and passing items across the midline to copying and drawing. |

## ACTIVITY AND TASK ANALYSIS

**Activity analysis** is the process that an OT uses to explore the demands of an activity and the range of skills needed to complete the task by breaking it into small steps in order to determine its therapeutic potential. It creates an understanding of what is needed to perform the activity so that the therapist can teach the patient how to complete the activity, and it determines the equipment, material, space, cost, and time required to perform the activity. **Task analysis** is the process in which a task is broken down into smaller, more manageable pieces that can be taught, practiced, and reinforced step by step, for example, walking into the kitchen, turning on the light, opening the fridge, gathering sandwich components, etc. **Grading** an activity is the modification of the activity to support the client's performance. Activities can be graded to make the task easier or more difficult, depending on the goal. Activities can be graded by increasing or decreasing the difficulty of a task by altering the number of steps or the complexity of the steps required to complete it, the amount of time given, or the amount or type of cues or assistance given during the activity.

## MET LEVELS

**Metabolic equivalent (MET) levels** describe the intensity and amount of energy that a person will use during an activity. One MET is the amount of energy that a person uses per unit of body weight during 1 minute of rest. MET levels are most often used in cardiac rehabilitation settings. Patients who have had a heart attack or heart surgery need to carefully work back into a typical and normal activity level. Therapists will use MET levels as a guide to ensure that the activity does not exceed what the patient's heart can tolerate during the healing process.

| MET | Intensity | Activity |
|---|---|---|
| 3 and under | Light activity | Sitting, reading, grooming, dressing, hygiene, crafts, and basic ADLs |
| 3–6 | Moderate aerobic activity | Walking briskly, hiking, dancing, housework, resistance exercises while sitting, up to 10 lbs. |
| 6 and above | Vigorous and intense aerobic activity | Running, competition sports, swimming |

## BORG RATING OF PERCEIVED EXERTION

The **Borg Rating of Perceived Exertion** is a scale that is used to measure how hard you feel like your body is working during physical activity. This scale allows therapists a reference point in order to grade tasks for patients to successfully complete tasks and attain goals.

| Exertion Description | Borg Rating | Examples (for most adults <65 years old) |
| --- | --- | --- |
| None | 6 | Reading a book, watching television |
| Very, very light | 7 to 8 | Tying shoes |
| Very light | 9 to 10 | Folding clothes |
| Fairly light | 11 to 12 | Walking through the grocery store |
| Somewhat hard | 13 to 14 | Brisk walking |
| Hard | 15 to 16 | Bicycling or swimming |
| Very hard | 17 to 18 | Highest level of sustained activity |
| Very, very hard | 19 to 20 | Finishing kick in a race |

## HAWAII EARLY LEARNING PROFILE

The **Hawaii Early Learning Profile** is not a standardized test, but a curriculum-based assessment used to identify needs, monitor growth and development, and create goals and a plan of care for treatment. It is an observation-based assessment for children birth to age 3 with an additional section for ages 3–6. It can take up to 90 minutes to administer the test. This test supports federal requirements for Part C of the Individuals with Disabilities Education Act and Early Head Start programs. The assessment is divided into seven domains: regulatory/sensory organization, cognitive, language, gross motor, fine motor, social-emotional, and self-help. Each domain is divided into strands, and each strand has a number to further specify the area. Domain 6.0 is self-help/behavioral skills, and strand 6.115 is putting both shoes correctly on each foot. Each of the strands is made up of skills, and each skill is built on the previous skill. The test is given at evaluation, monthly during treatment, and again at discharge or transition through the system. The test is scored as a (+) if the skill is present, a (–) if the skill is not present, a (+/–) if the skill is emerging, and as a (N/A) if it is not applicable.

## BI

The **Barthel index (BI)** is a standardized test that uses an ordinal scale to rate a patient's ability to complete self-care and mobility in ADLs. The BI was one of the first standardized tools to assess ADLs, and the FIM was created to be a more comprehensive test based on the BI. The goal is to determine the level of independence that each patient has without the use of verbal or physical help or cues. It assesses levels of independence in 10 ADL tasks with a score range of 0 (dependent) to 20 (independent). These areas include dressing, feeding, grooming, toileting, bathing, bed/chair transfers, walking, stairs, bladder, and bowels. With a score of greater than 85, the patient will likely reintegrate into the community independently and could live alone. A score of less than 40 would indicate significant deficits in ADLs and mobility, and the patient would be unlikely to return home and would need 24/7 care.

**Score = Level of Disability**
0– 20 = Total dependence
21– 60 = Severe dependence
61– 90 = Moderate dependence
91– 99 = Slight dependence
100 = Independence

## SFA

The **School Function Assessment (SFA)** is a standardized criterion-referenced assessment that measures school-related functional skills of elementary school children grades K–6. The assessment is completed by one or multiple school professionals (therapist, teacher, etc.) that see the child regularly and can observe the child during activity; it can take several days to administer. The SFA has three components: participation, task supports, and activity performance. In the participation section of the test, the student is observed interacting in six areas: general or special education classroom, playground or recess, transportation to and from school, bathroom and toileting activities, transitions to and from class, and mealtime or snack time. Participation in each setting is scored on a 6-point scale with 1 being participation extremely limited and 6 being full participation. The task section looks at support being given to the student during tasks. The task support has four areas:

1. physical task support: assistance
2. physical task support: adaptations
3. cognitive/behavioral task support: assistance
4. cognitive/behavioral task support: adaptations.

Supports are measured on a 4-point scale with 1 being extensive assistance or adaptations and 4 being no assistance or adaptations. The activity performance section addresses travel, maintaining and changing position, recreational movement, manipulation with movement, using materials, setup and cleanup, eating and drinking, hygiene, clothing management, functional communication, memory and understanding, following social conventions, compliance with adult directives and school rules, task behavior/completion, positive interaction, behavior regulation, personal care awareness, and safety. This is measured on a 4-point scale with 1 being does not perform and 4 being performs consistently.

## ACLS

The **Allen Cognitive Level Screen (ACLS)** is a standardized screening assessment of functional cognition developed within the framework of the cognitive disabilities model by OT Claudia Allen. The patient's learning and problem-solving abilities are evaluated during the performance of three visual motor tasks of increasing complexity. The screen consists of learning three visual-motor tasks using leather-lacing stitches, and it can be completed in 20 minutes. This test was developed for use with adults with psychiatric disorders and dementia. The patient is tasked to complete three stitches: the running stitch, the whipstitch, and the cordovan stitch. Scores are numbers that correspond to the specific levels of supervision and care that are needed to function in daily life. Scores range from a low of 3.0 to a high of 5.8 and can indicate the need for 24/7 supervision for safety to complete independence and the ability to learn new tasks.

### ROUTINE TASK INVENTORY

The **Routine Task Inventory** is a part of the Allen Battery group of tools along with the ACLS developed within the framework of the cognitive disabilities model by OT Claudia Allen. It is an evidence-based, semi standardized assessment that looks at how the degree of cognitive disability interferes with everyday tasks using observation of task behavior. The therapist needs to observe the patient completing a minimum of four tasks from each area citing specifics about the task and duration of the activity. These areas include physical ADL, community IADL, communication, and work readiness. It can take several days to complete this assessment. Scores are associated with the Allen Scale of cognitive Levels 1–6, and a mean score is calculated for each subscale.

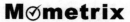

## KELS ASSESSMENT

The **Kohlman Evaluation of Living Skills (KELS)** is a standardized assessment used to determine the safety of a patient when reintegrating into the community to live independently. It is a criterion-based assessment that covers 13 living skills in the following 5 main areas: self-care, safety and health, money management, transportation and telephone, and work and leisure activity. Each section of the KELS is divided into method, equipment, administration procedures, and scoring. Items are scored as the patient being independent or needs assistance. The KELS is most often used to assess the senior population or patients post stroke or traumatic brain injury (TBI) in a rehabilitation or SNF setting, but it can be used on any patient from adolescent to late adulthood. It takes approximately 45 minutes to complete the assessment. The test is somewhat outdated with the last update performed in the early 1990s, so the pictures are dated and the Internet as a source is not addressed, so using options other than a phone book to find telephone numbers and writing a check for paying bills are key components of the assessment.

## COGNITIVE EVALUATIONS

**Cognitive testing** often falls under the job description of the OT, but it can also be completed by a speech therapist depending on the setting. It is always a good idea to discuss the cognitive evaluations that you choose with the speech therapist on staff because often both disciplines will test cognition to address different concerns and this ensures that you are not both using and administering the same assessment.

- **Saint Louis University Mental Status (SLUMS) Exam:** Evaluates attention and concentration, executive functions, memory, language, visuoconstructional skills, conceptual thinking, calculations, and orientation. It looks for cognitive deficits and cognition changes over time. It is norm-standardized and used in all settings. There are 11 items in the exam, and scores will indicate normal cognitive function, mild neurocognitive disorder, or dementia.
- **Mini-Mental State Examination:** Evaluates orientation, registration, attention, calculation, and language and praxis. It is norm-standardized and used in all settings. There are 30 questions on the exam with scores indicating normal cognitive function, mild cognitive impairment, moderate cognitive impairment, and severe cognitive impairment.
- **Short Blessed Test**: Evaluates cognitive concerns in the areas of orientation, memory, and concentration to determine cognitive changes associated with dementia. It is norm-standardized and used in all settings. There are six items on the exam, and the scores will indicate normal cognitive function, minimum impairment, minimal to moderate impairment, and severe impairment.
- **Montreal Cognitive Assessment:** Evaluates the ability to process and understand visual information, executive function, language, short-term memory recall, attention, concentration, working memory, and awareness of time and place. It is norm-standardized and used in all settings. There are 16 items in 8 categories on the exam, and scores will indicate mild cognitive impairment and Alzheimer's disease.

## GLASGOW COMA SCALE

The **Glasgow Coma Scale** is a neurological scale used to determine the level of consciousness in a brain-injured or comatose patient. The test measures the motor response, verbal response, and eye-opening response in a patient.

| Behavior | Response | Score |
|---|---|---|
| Eye opening | Spontaneously | 4 |
| | To speech | 3 |

52

| Behavior | Response | Score |
|---|---|---|
|  | To pain | 2 |
|  | No response | 1 |
| **Best verbal** | Oriented to time, place, and person | 5 |
|  | Confused | 4 |
|  | Inappropriate words | 3 |
|  | Incomprehensible sounds | 2 |
|  | No response | 1 |
| **Best motor** | Obeys commands | 6 |
|  | Moves to localized pain | 5 |
|  | Flexion withdrawal from pain | 4 |
|  | Abnormal flexion (decorticate) | 3 |
|  | Abnormal extension (decerebrate) | 2 |
|  | No response | 1 |
| **Total score:** | Best response | **15** |
|  | Comatose client | **8 or less** |
|  | Totally Unresponsive | **3** |

## RANCHO LOS AMIGOS SCALE

The **Rancho Los Amigos Scale (RLAS)** is also a neurological scale and it is used to assess individuals after a closed head injury and is based on cognitive and behavioral presentations as they emerge from their coma. It tracks the levels of awareness, cognition, behavior and interaction with the environment.

| Level | Response | Assistance Needed? |
|---|---|---|
| I | None | Total |
| II | Generalized | Total |
| III | Localized | Total |
| IV | Confused-Agitated | Maximal |
| V | Confused-Inappropriate | Maximal |
| VI | Confused-Appropriate | Moderate |
| VII | Automatic-Appropriate | Minimal |
| VIII | Purposeful-Appropriate | Stand-By |

## COMMON WRIST FRACTURES

In an outpatient clinic, much of the occupational therapy caseload will be made up of hand injuries and UE deficits, even if the therapist is not a certified hand therapist. These are the most common injuries and interventions seen in a clinic. Treatment interventions for wrist fractures will include but are not limited to the wrist generally being in a cast for 6–8 weeks prior to therapy. On assessment when the cast is removed, there is a possible need for splinting to further immobilize or for pain management. The patient's ROM, strength, sensation, dexterity, and edema are assessed. A functional activity assessment is completed. Treatment sessions would include physical agent modalities (PAMs); pain management; edema and wound management; retrograde and scar massage; fine motor; dexterity; strength; monitoring of the neck, shoulder, and elbow for pain or stiffness; active assistive and passive ROM; and modification and task analysis of the home, workplace, and ADLs. The following are common wrist fractures seen in a clinic:

| Wrist Fracture | Definition |
|---|---|
| Colles' fracture | Caused when a person falls and tries to catch themselves with the wrist extended. The distal part of the radius breaks causing it to point in a dorsal direction. |
| Smith's fracture | A "reverse Colles' fracture," which is caused by falling on a flexed wrist or an impact to the dorsal forearm causing the distal part of the radius to point in a ventral direction. |
| Distal radius fracture | Caused by falling with the arms extended when a person is trying to catch themselves. A Colles' fracture is the most common type of radial fracture. Distal radial fractures can be intra-articular or extra-articular. In an intra-articular fracture, the broken piece of the radius extends into the joint, whereas in an extra-articular fracture, the broken part of the radius does not extend into the joint itself. |
| Barton's fracture | Caused by falling on an extended and pronated wrist. A Barton's fracture is a distal radius fracture with a dislocation of the radiocarpal joint. It can be dorsal or palmar. These are most often surgically repaired with an open reduction and internal fixation. |
| Scaphoid fracture | A break in the scaphoid bone, which is the carpal bone at the base of the thumb. This is most often injured when you fall on the palm of your extended hand. |
| Distal ulna fracture | These injuries are seen at the distal end of the ulna where the radius and ulna articulate with the bone in the wrist. This is usually not an independent fracture and is seen in addition to a distal radius fracture. It is usually injured when there is too much rotation of the wrist or an extreme force against the ulna. There is most often a significant ligament injury as well. |

## TYPES OF BONE FRACTURES

A bone fracture is caused when the force against the bone is greater than the bone can sustain causing it to splinter, fracture, or break. There are multiple classifications of fractures. A **closed fracture** is when the bone breaks but does not puncture through the skin and protrude through to the outside. An **open fracture** is when the bone breaks and punctures the skin protruding to the outside of the body. A **comminuted fracture** is when the bone breaks in multiple areas. This is often seen in a trauma such as a car accident or in competitive sports. A **greenstick fracture** is when part of the bone bends and does not fully break. This is often seen in young children because the bones are flexible, softer, and still developing. A **spiral fracture** is when the bone is twisted or rotated like a corkscrew. An **avulsion fracture** is when a tendon or ligament is taxed and pulled too hard causing it to pull away and break the bone. An **oblique fracture** is a break at an angle caused by the outside force coming at a right angle to the bone. A **transverse fracture** is when the fracture is perpendicular to the shaft of the bone. A **pathological fracture** is caused by disease making the bone weak, and the bone can break without warning simply by putting minimal pressure on it.

## COMMON TENDON AND NERVE INJURIES

Tendon and nerve injuries can be a result of disease, trauma, and surgery. This can be because the structure itself has been cut, overstretched, crushed, pinched, or compressed. When there is damage to the tendons and nerves in the hand, a patient can lose sensation and the ability to move the wrist functionally either due to wrist drop or inability to extend the wrist as well as compromised muscle tone in the shoulder, arms, and hand affecting functional movement and ADLs. Patients also often complain of pain, numbness, tingling, and hypersensitivity. Therapeutic treatment will likely include splinting, PAMs, vibration and sensory modalities, tendon gliding exercises, environmental modification, adaptive equipment, edema and pain management, wound care if there was surgery, establishing a home exercise program, fine motor and dexterity activities, ROM exercises, and exercises that will increase the use of the hand and UE. These are the most common injuries seen in a clinic. The following are common tendon and nerve injuries seen in a clinic:

| Injury | Definition |
| --- | --- |
| Carpal tunnel syndrome | The carpal tunnel is the narrow area in the volar wrist where tendons, ligaments, and nerves pass to provide sensation and mobility in the hand and fingers. Carpal tunnel syndrome is when the median nerve is compressed causing numbness, tingling, and pain. Often seen with repetitive hand movement such as with frequent computer use. Often, a carpal tunnel release is surgically completed prior to therapy. |
| Flexor tendon injury | Flexor tendons are found on the volar side of the hand and are superficial to the skin. They are responsible for bending the fingers. Injury is caused when the tendon is pulled out of the sheath and away from the bone by physical sports, diseases such as RA, or a deep cut to the palm or fingers. |
| Extensor tendon injury | Extensor tendons are found on the dorsal side of the hand and are superficial to the skin. They are responsible for extending the fingers. Injury is caused when the tendon is pulled out of the sheath and away from the bone by physical sports when the finger gets jammed, diseases such as RA, or a superficial cut to the back of the hand. The most common types are a mallet finger/baseball finger (extreme force causing flexion, such as jamming the finger when catching a ball) or boutonniere deformity (the finger is bent at the PIP joint, or the thumb is bent at the DIP joint caused by tendon injury or RA). |
| Radial nerve damage | The radial nerve is responsible for sensation on the dorsum of the hand and extension of the fingers and wrist for assisting in functional grasp. Damage is caused by physical trauma or infection. |
| Ulnar nerve damage | The ulnar nerve is responsible for sensation of the ring and pinkie fingers and fine motor control of the hand. Damage is often caused by elbow injury, nerve trauma, infection, and increased edema. |
| Median nerve damage | The median nerve is responsible for sensation on the thumb, middle, and ring fingers and flexion of the fingers and thumb for assisting in functional grasp. Most often, damage is related to carpal tunnel injury, but it can also be caused by trauma, edema, and infection. |

## ORTHOPEDIC INTERVENTION FOR TOTAL KNEE REPLACEMENT

There are two types of knee replacement surgeries: **total knee replacement (TKR)** and **partial knee replacement (PKR)**. TKR, or total knee arthroplasty (TKA), is a surgical procedure in which parts of the knee joint are replaced with artificial parts (prosthetic). In a PKR, the damaged portion of the knee (bone and/or cartilage) is replaced with metal and plastic components. The need for these surgeries can be because of trauma or arthritic issues. A TKR is more commonly seen than a PKR. Generally, people are up and walking hours after surgery and will be **weight-bearing as tolerated** barring any complications, and patients can put as much weight as they can tolerate on the surgical knee. In the hospital, the OT will evaluate the patient's ability to care for themselves at home including getting in and out of bed, functional transfers, toileting, self-care, dressing, and grooming and will review the equipment needed for the return home post-surgery (shower chair, toilet riser or commode, reacher, sock aide, and long-handled shoehorn). The home health or facility-based (SNF or rehab) OT will further address using the stairs, getting in and out of the car, meal prep, laundry, dressing techniques, energy conservation, as well as UE strengthening because there will likely be more emphasis on arms for transfers and activity while the LE recovers and heals.

## ORTHOPEDIC INTERVENTIONS FOR TOTAL HIP REPLACEMENT

A **total hip replacement or total hip arthroplasty** is the surgical removal of the ball and socket and replacement with a metal ball and stem inserted into the femur bone and an artificial cup socket. Surgical approaches can be completed by surgically entering posteriorly or anteriorly, and each approach will require different precautions for the patient. In a **posterior approach**, the patient will be unable to bend at the hip past a 90-degree angle, cross their legs, or twist the hip inward (pigeon toe). In an **anterior approach**, the patient is not allowed to step backwards with the surgical leg into hip extension, externally rotate the surgical leg, cross their legs, sleep on the surgical side in a side-lying position, and must use a pillow to support a neutral hip when rolling in bed. These precautions are generally in place for 4-8 weeks depending on the surgeon. The main goal of the hospital OT is to reinforce hip precautions while completing ADLs. The OT will evaluate the patient's ability to care for themselves at home including getting in and out of bed, functional transfers, toileting, self-care, dressing, and grooming and will review the equipment needed for return home post-surgery such as a shower chair, toilet riser, or commode. The therapist will also educate the patient in the use of a hip kit, which contains a reacher, sock aid, long-handled shoehorn, and long-handled sponge. The home health or facility-based (SNF or rehab) OT will teach the more advanced ADL skills while continuing to enforce hip precautions.

## ORTHOPEDIC INTERVENTIONS FOR TOTAL SHOULDER ARTHROPLASTY

A **total shoulder arthroplasty** is the surgical removal of the ball and socket and replacement with a metal ball and stem inserted into the humeral bone and an artificial cup socket. The need for this surgery can be caused by arthritis, fracture or trauma, or a rotator cuff repair. Post-surgery, the patient will likely wear a sling for 4–6 weeks, only taking it off for exercise and ADL activity, and will be told to not participate in activities that require active movement and pushing or pulling of the surgical arm. Each surgeon will likely have his/her own protocols based on the surgery techniques used, and therapy is guided by the specific ROM designated by the surgeon. The hospital OT will be tasked with teaching how to don/doff the sling and sling care, teaching one-handed ADL techniques, and in most cases only hand, wrist, and elbow ROM and pendulum exercises. Facility and home health therapists will continue refining single-arm ADLs including dressing, bathing, and cooking. At the 6- to 8-week mark, patients will generally begin seeing an outpatient therapist to begin work on strengthening and ROM and start to return to full and normal functioning.

## IMPORTANCE OF OCCUPATIONAL THERAPY IN HEALTH LITERACY

According to the Department of Health and Human Services, **health literacy** is the "ability of the individual to access, understand, and use health-related information and services to make appropriate health decisions." Healthcare professionals often recommend treatments and activities for the overall health of a patient that are complex and not easily understood for a nonmedical or uneducated person. The average American reads at a sixth-grade level, and with the influx of patients with English as a second language, the ever-changing healthcare system becomes more difficult to navigate for the average person. OTs are unique in that they are skilled in task analysis and are adept at deconstructing tasks and information to a level that is understandable for their patients. If a patient is instructed by their physician to "eat healthier" after having a heart attack, does the patient understand what this means? The OT can identify that the person does not understand what "eating healthy" means and can break the task down into understanding food labels, shopping the outside perimeter of the grocery store for fresh products, and identifying correct portion sizes. The OT can create a therapy session around making a shopping list, gathering the items at the store, and prepping and cooking a healthy meal.

## STANDARDIZED ASSESSMENTS ADD TO THE VALIDITY OF THE PROFESSION

A **standardized test** is defined as a test that:

- can be administered, scored, and interpreted in a consistent manner without bias
- can be duplicated
- can be given in diverse settings
- will compare function and ability across a variety of populations

Standardized tests are considered a fair and objective method of assessing skills, without bias, and there is room for interpretation by the provider of the test. They provide a good measure of a patient's ability, which demonstrates credibility, and they justify that the therapy interventions that are provided actually work. With the profession as a whole moving toward a focus of evidence-based practice, standardized testing is not only needed, but it is crucial to the support and justification of intervention and validating the need for services. Currently, as well as into the foreseeable future, reimbursement from our continually changing healthcare system will become increasingly reliant upon occupational therapy services to demonstrate patient progress through documented, accurate, and reliable testing.

## MULTIDISCIPLINARY TEAM IN HEALTHCARE

A **multidisciplinary team** is when a group of medical professionals come together to work for the betterment and success of the patient's healthcare needs with a collaborative approach. This is how a patient can have the most comprehensive medical treatment possible because the different disciplines' scopes of practice work to complement each other, meeting all of the patient's concerns in a more thorough manner to create the best outcome. A team approach allows for the patient's physical, social, and emotional needs to be met. In addition to creating better outcomes for the patient, studies are beginning to show that a team approach allows for more checks and balances to prevent adverse events and higher patient satisfaction. Teams vary based on the setting, but they can include physicians, nurses, aides, floor directors/unit directors, PTs, OTs, speech-language pathologists (SLPs), dietary/nutritionists, social workers, case managers, psychiatrists/psychologists, and pharmacists. The therapists on the team (PT, OT, SLP) will typically have a unique and important role because they will have more frequent and daily interactions with the patient than the other members of the team. Often, it is these therapists that notice more subtle changes or concerns because they are treating the patient for 45 minutes or longer every day whereas other staff see the patient briefly each day, only once a week, or because of shift work they will have multiple days off between interactions with the patient.

## CARE COORDINATION MEETINGS IN HEALTHCARE

A **care coordination meeting** is a meeting to discuss each patient's care, progress, and discharge planning on a weekly basis. These meeting will have various members based on the setting, but they most often include a case manager, therapy nurse, and physician. The focus is determining the length of stay, assessing readmission risk, discussing barriers to discharge (help at home, independence with mobility, and ADLs), discharge locations (home, SNF, rehabilitation center), equipment needs (oxygen, walker, commode) and current concerns, family and patient questions, patient education, family training, and complications or complaints. Therapy plays a pivotal role because it is the therapist who determines safety and independence with mobility and self-care and has a strong influence on the safest location for discharge. Additionally, in a skilled nursing setting, the care coordination meeting will discuss Medicare and insurance coverage days and the patient's

57

utilization group (RUG) level, which is a classification system to determine
...oursement levels for patients in SNFs.

## STANDARDS OF PRACTICE

The term **standards of practice** in occupational therapy is the baseline and minimum standard
needed to be a practicing therapist as defined by the American Occupational Therapy Association
(AOTA). It is a combination of skills, knowledge, understanding, ethics, and responsibilities. The
first and most important rule is that all OTs and occupational therapy assistants must practice
under the rules and guidelines of federal and state laws. This means that the therapist has
graduated from an occupational therapy program accredited by the Accreditation Council for
Occupational Therapy Education (ACOTE), has completed fieldwork requirements, has passed the
national testing through the National Board for Certification in Occupational Therapy (NBCOT), and
has a state license in the state they are working in. Additionally, there are four standard areas that
must be met: (1) professional standing and responsibility, (2) screening, evaluation, and
reevaluation, (3) intervention, and (4) outcomes. The AOTA "Standards of Practice for Occupational
Therapy" was last updated in 2010 and is available at AOTA.org.

## IMPACT OF KEY LEGISLATION ON THERAPY SERVICES

Legislation can have a major effect on the treatment of your patients, and it is important to stay
abreast of new rules and laws throughout your career. The American Occupational Therapy
Association (AOTA) website is always the most up to date with current laws and regulations.

| Statute/Act | Content |
| --- | --- |
| Rehabilitation Act of 1973 (Section 504) | The Rehabilitation Act is a federal statute created to protect people with disabilities from discrimination based on their disability. Section 504 requires schools to meet the needs of students with disabilities in the same that they would for children with no special needs. Accommodations can include extended time on tests or assignments, adaptive equipment, alternative and flexible seating, behavioral or educational contracts, and peer-to-peer counseling or teacher aides. |
| Americans with Disabilities Act of 1990 (ADA) | The Americans with Disabilities Act (ADA) is a civil rights law that protects people with disabilities against discrimination in all areas of life. This includes all areas open to the general public in public and private businesses, schools, parks, places of employment, and public transportation. |
| Individuals with Disabilities Education Act of 1997 | This act states that every child has a right to free and appropriate education and states that children with disabilities can be educated with their nondisabled peers. It requires every state to have policies and procedures in place and allows for assistive technology for children ages 3 to 21. |
| Assistive Technology Act of 1998 | Provides state funding for assistive technology through programming to ensure that technology-related assistance and devices are available for people with disabilities. |
| The Developmental Disabilities Assistance and Bill of Rights Act of 2000 | Provides grants, protection, and advocacy groups for people with developmental disabilities including funding for university-based and affiliated programming. |

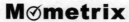

## CREATING A TREATMENT PLAN AND DOCUMENTING GOALS

A treatment plan is the key part of the initial evaluation process. The evaluation of a patient can be separated into three parts: (1) background information, history, and physical, (2) assessments and testing, and (3) the treatment plan. A **treatment plan** is a combination of short- and long-term goals; treatment procedures and activity; amount, duration, frequency and anticipated number of visits; and recommendations including discharge equipment and referrals. The plan must have input from the patient and demonstrate evidence and need for the therapy intervention. **Goals** are established by determining what tasks the patient wants to be able to participate in, what is causing the patient to be unable to complete the task, and how that task can be made possible and attainable. Goals should always be functional, measurable, observable, and attainable in a reasonable amount of time. In most settings there will be **short-term goals (STGs)** and **long-term goals (LTGs)**. STGs are directly related to LTGs and are the building blocks and often the individual performance components of LTGs. LTGs are the activities and skills that the patient and therapist would like to see the patient master by the time of discharge from treatment.

## PROGRESS NOTES AND DISCHARGE REPORTS

A **progress note** is written for each therapy session and is a description of the treatment intervention and the patient response to that treatment. It will also include the start and end time, a progress indicator with regard to the stated goals (if the patient is progressing toward established goals), documentation of pain, and plans and recommendations. A signature from the therapist makes it a legal document. Progress notes can be narrative or in SOAP note form, and they must be clear, consistent, and accurate with the treatment activity. Often, a more detailed exercise log will be attached to the progress note with specific exercises and activities detailed with the amount of weights used or the time needed to complete the activity and number of repetitions. The goal of the progress note is that any therapist could step in and provide and continue treatment that is in line with the plan of care in place and to keep a detailed chronological log of patient progress and success. A **discharge summary** is completed at the discontinuation of therapy services. It summarizes the therapy sessions, addresses progress toward goals, and makes recommendations. A discharge report will include identifying information in detail (name, age, diagnosis, and precautions), date of evaluation, and discharge with the number of visits, interventions and modalities that were used, summary of goals and their progress, standardized testing results, and recommendations. Again, the document must be signed by the therapist to make it a legal document.

## DOCUMENTATION TECHNIQUES

**Documentation** of therapy encounters is a significant part of the day for a working therapist. Documentation is required for every therapy session and must follow the rules established by the facility and regulatory organizations. Most documentation is electronic, but some facilities are still using handwritten notes. All handwritten entries are to be written in blue ink and will include original signatures. This is to easily identify an original note and not a copy of the original. Notes can be written in SOAP format or as narrative notes. SOAP stands for subjective, objective, assessment, and plan. A narrative note is a description of the therapy session documenting the sequence of events as they happened making sure to identify as much specific and descriptive information as possible.

| S | Subjective: Document what the patient states are the limitations, concerns, problems, and deficits. |
|---|---|
| O | Objective: Document all measurable, observable, and quantifiable data. |
| A | Assessment: Document the professional opinion and judgment regarding patient limits and strengths, goals and barriers, progress, and rehabilitation potential. |
| P | Plan: Document ongoing plan to reach the goals established at evaluation. |

## EARLY INTERVENTION PROGRAMMING

**Early intervention programming** is a service provided by the government for children from birth to the age of 2 with developmental delays or specific health conditions or diagnoses in order to help them catch up in reaching developmental milestones to be successful in school and eventually become a functional member of society. Services are delivered at no or low cost to the child and are provided under the Individuals with Disabilities Education Act (IDEA). Under IDEA Part C, occupational therapy is considered a primary service, which means that the OT can be the only service provider the child has or can act as a service coordinator or member of an evaluation team. As a service coordinator, the OT provides client-centered, occupation-based services to the child and family by encouraging bonding between the child and family, educating the family, promoting achievement of milestones, patterning routines and play, adapting the environment so the child is successful with tasks, and encouraging the family to be advocates for their child. As a service coordinator, the OT can assist the family through the Part C early intervention assessment, intervention, and transition process.

## DETERMINING THE FREQUENCY AND DURATION OF INTERVENTION

The frequency and duration of services are based on the setting of practice and clinical judgment. Frequency is the amount of times each week/month that the patient will be seen, and the duration is for how long in total. Clinical judgment determined by the evaluating therapist is always the number-one factor, and it is based on patient activity tolerance, progression of illness or disability, new skill acquisition ability, or the ability to recover lost or impaired skills. Outside factors that influence duration can include hospital or facility length of stay, insurance authorization for number of sessions, RUG levels, and the patient's ability to meet the copay. According to the AOTA code of ethics, it is a violation to continue to treat a patient who is no longer benefiting from therapy. The therapist must discharge the patient when the therapy provided does not meet the goals and services of the patient or when progress can't be shown in a measurable outcome. Services should be terminated when the patient is no longer making progress and has met the highest level of functional potential and is unwilling or unable to continue working and meeting their goals.

## HEPs

A **home exercise program (HEP)** is a series of exercises or activities created by the therapist in order to provide continued training and activity outside of the scheduled therapy sessions. Treatment is almost always supplemented with the construction of a HEP to allow for carryover of treatment principles into the home setting as appropriate. This can be simple UE or LE exercises against gravity or with a TheraBand for strength and endurance, fine motor or dexterity exercises with putty for a hand injury or stroke, or task-related activities such as folding towels or making a sandwich. A well-designed HEP will help the patient build on the skills learned in each therapy session so that progression to new activities and tasks can be addressed in each session.

## IEPs

An **Individualized Education Plan (IEP)** is a document that is created for children ages 3 to 21 who need special education services. The IEP establishes guidelines and goals based on federal regulations to accommodate and assist a child who has an established and documented physical, cognitive, or learning disability. The document is created and updated yearly by the child's teachers, therapists, and other paraprofessionals with input from the family, and there is a yearly team meeting to discuss the child's progress and update goals. The IEP remains in place through the child's high school graduation or 21st birthday. The goal is to assist the child to be as successful as possible in school and in their academic career. The role of the OT is to address the impact that the disability has on the child's ability to function and participate in the educational process as successfully as possible.

## WORKER HEALTH PROGRAMS

In the outpatient setting, a therapist will likely see many workers' compensation and workplace injury patients. When someone is injured at work, they are frequently sent to therapy to address the injury and functional deficits that are keeping them for their jobs. Treatment sessions will include work simulation activities and strengthening and conditioning activities to get injured workers back to work as quickly as possible. The facility may also have a contract with local businesses to complete work readiness evaluations during a preemployment screening. Screens and evaluations may include a **functional capacity evaluation**, which is a standardized and peer-reviewed evaluation tool that measures strength, endurance, physical demand, work level, and positional tolerance. This may be done preemployment, or it can be used to determine return-to-work status including identifying if a patient can return to full duty or needs to return with modified or transitional duty. **Work hardening** is a program designed to return the employee to work by completing activities that include real or simulated work activities in line with their job. The goal is to improve and restore physical, behavioral, and vocational functions so that the person can return to active duty at his or her place of employment. **Work conditioning** is more general and goal oriented to address deficits in strength, endurance, ROM, joint mobility, and functional abilities with the same intent: to get a patient returned to full duty at work.

## GROUP TREATMENT

OTs have been using groups since the beginning of the profession in order to facilitate learning and support positive interactions. **Group treatment** is task and activity based and is used for enhancing and mastering skills; increasing strength or physical ability; and increasing comradery, communication, and social skills while recovering from illness or injury. There are many benefits to running groups for occupational therapy interventions. Groups are often seen in mental health settings using trust- and team-building activities, as well as simulated role play to elicit increased communication skills, emotional regulation, appropriate social interactions, and teamwork among group members. In pediatric settings, children can be seen in groups to foster appropriate interactions between children and to initiate play strategies and self-regulation. Groups with parents and children are often used so that therapists can assist the parents in modeling appropriate behaviors and interacting in public with multiple sensory inputs. In a rehabilitation setting, groups often include ADL groups, exercise groups, family training, and teaching patients how to use adaptive devices and electronics.

## MONITORING THE EFFECTIVENESS IN A GROUP INTERVENTION

The key to the success of any **group intervention** is monitoring the success and failures of the group throughout the activity. Monitoring allows the program to determine what is and is not working so that adjustments can be made to keep the group successful and on task as well as

61

continue to establish the need and importance of the group. Frequent monitoring can encompass standardized testing, surveys, the ability of the members to participate and finish tasks, and member exit interviews. This allows the group leaders to see what is actually happening in the group versus what the group had planned to accomplish. The ability to show the success of a group through frequent monitoring can also impact funding including the ability to apply for and maintain grants.

## SCOPE OF PRACTICE VS. AREAS OF PRACTICE

The occupational therapy **scope of practice** is the domain and process of what a therapist is allowed to do. **Domain** can be defined as the occupation that the patient finds meaning in during their everyday life. The **process** of occupational therapy is specifically the delivery of service within occupational therapy. These activities include evaluation, testing, goals, interventions, and final outcomes. The OT is responsible for all of the treatment as well as the safety and effectiveness of the treatment and the modalities. A certified occupational therapy assistant (COTA) can provide occupational therapy services under the supervision and license of the OT based on the treatment goals and interventions designated by the OT during the evaluation process. According to AOTA, there are six main **areas of practice** for an OT. Within each setting, there is unlimited potential to find areas that interest you and create your own niche or job. These six areas include children and youth, mental health, health and wellness, work and industry, productive aging, and rehabilitation and disability.

## IMPORTANCE OF PROGRAM DESIGN AND DEVELOPMENT

An OT is not limited to traditional settings or areas of practice. Many therapists see a need in their facility or in the community that could be addressed by therapy to meet the needs of a large population. It can be something as simple as a balance and exercise program to prevent falls in a senior center or a modified swim class for children with special needs at the local community center. Once the idea is born, a plan with specific details of the program activities, resource allocations and financial needs, and expected outcomes of the program needs to be documented to present to the community or organization. Program design has the potential to create areas of practice outside of the traditional hospital or clinic settings and create an impact on a larger portion of the population that may not be reached by traditional therapeutic approaches.

## UPDATING A PLAN OF CARE

A **plan of care (POC)** is the therapy document that is a written and signed plan of the patient's care establishing the diagnoses, treatment goals, treatment modalities, and interventions and the amount, duration, and frequency of therapy services. This is written and signed by the evaluating therapist and then submitted to the physician or nurse practitioner for approval. Progress notes are created on the 10th treatment day or the 30th calendar day of the episode of treatment and are submitted to the treating physician. At this time, updates are generally made to the POC based on the patients' progress. Standardized testing is completed to determine if progress has been made since the initial evaluation and to address if the goals have been met or if the patient is progressing on the goals, and the therapist needs to determine the effectiveness of the overall therapy interventions including if the patient has met their highest level of functional potential and if there are still skills that need to be achieved. This is all documented and submitted to the physician for sign-off. Although the POC is most often updated during the progress note, it can be altered and changed at any time during the therapy process if the therapist feels that the goals are not appropriate, the patient's medical status has changed, or the frequency needs to be updated.

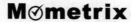

## DETERMINING ELIGIBILITY FOR SERVICES

Determining eligibility for services is the key for reimbursement with insurance companies and Medicare, and it is based on medical necessity. **Medical necessity** refers to healthcare services that a therapist provides using clinical judgment that would allow a patient to be successful in managing, treating, or recovering from an illness, injury, or a disease and its symptoms. When medical necessity is established, the patient's insurance will determine eligibility. This is usually based on if therapy services will improve or restore functional ability or prevent the patient from getting worse. Once a physician has initiated a referral for therapy, it is up to the therapist to document and justify need. In the initial evaluation, the therapist needs to show that the judgment, knowledge, and skills of a licensed therapist are required to prevent the worsening of a condition; improve, correct, or cure a symptom or condition; increase function; or decrease the deficits resulting from a documented dysfunction. Throughout treatment, the therapist needs to continue to justify need by documenting a clear picture of the treatment sessions including progress on goals, updates to the plan of care, and the direction in which the treatment is heading on the road to discharge from service.

## MAINTENANCE AND RESTORATIVE THERAPY PROGRAMS

A **maintenance program** is a program that is created by a therapist toward the end of the therapy sessions in order to maintain functional status and prevent decline with discharge from services. Maintenance programs can also be established after the therapist completes a "screen" on a patient in order to address a resident's ability to maintain their functional status or the patient is at risk for functional decline. Screens are often completed in long-term-care and assisted-living facilities. A **screen** is a nonbillable treatment intervention to look at strength, ROM, and flexibility as well as functional ability and cognition. It is usually initiated by an incident such as a fall or by staff noticing a decline in functional ability. The screen will determine the need for therapeutic evaluation and intervention or the need for the patient to be on a restorative or maintenance program. A **restorative therapy program** is a program established by the therapist to prevent decline after the patient has been discharged from therapy services. It is activities, exercises, and tasks created by the therapist and run by nursing assistants or nonclinical therapy staff. Activities can include transfers, bed mobility exercises, fine motor tasks, and functional mobility. Restorative therapy aids are in most cases trained by and signed off on by the treating therapist.

## MAXIMIZING SAFETY IN THE CARE DELIVERY OR SERVICES

Therapy treatments are fluid in nature. Therapists enter a session with a plan in place with the activity and skills that they plan to address each session. However, when treating a living, breathing person, sessions can change quickly for many reasons. A patient can have a medical emergency or be emotionally unstable on any given day, and this can change throughout the session. Therapists needs to be aware of signs that can indicate a physical problem such as diaphoresis, skin pallor, attention levels, and breathing. Additionally, nonverbal signs of aggression and psychosocial issues such as tensions with guests and family members can affect therapy and patient and therapist safety. Being aware of how to get help quickly, the ability to cotreat for patient and therapist safety, and changing tasks quickly to promote safety are important skills as a therapist. Safe patient handling and mobility refers to policies and program interventions that direct how healthcare professionals move patients in a way that does not cause strain or injury to the patient to themselves. Most facilities have their own specific guidelines including items such as manual lifting of patients becoming minimized and encouraging the use of a mechanical lifts, ergonomic training for transfers and mobility, and creating strengthening programs for staff to address their own stress, strength, and body fatigue.

# Intervention Management

## ISOLATION PRECAUTIONS

People are placed in **isolation precautions** in order to prevent cross-transmission or cross-infection. In most facilities, patients with these infections will still be seen by a therapist, but the therapist will need to use personal protective equipment such as gowns, gloves, foot and eye protection, and masks. The following infections are commonly seen in healthcare and require isolation precautions:

- **Cellulitis**: A bacterial skin infection. It usually only affects the surface of the skin, but it can impact the blood and lymph nodes if the bacteria enter through a cut on the skin. The skin gets hot, red, swollen, and painful in the affected area. It is usually seen in the lower extremities and is not airborne.
- **Methicillin-resistant *Staphylococcus aureus***: A type of staph infection that is resistant to most antibiotics, which is why it is sometimes called a superbug. It is spread by direct contact to a wound or by touching dirty hands. It can cause skin infection, pneumonia, or sepsis if it gets into the bloodstream through a wound. Often it first presents as a bump or rash that is misinterpreted as a spider bite. It is only airborne if in the lungs.
- ***Klebsiella pneumoniae***: Bacteria that live in the intestines that can be problematic if they move to other places. Has the potential to turn into a superbug because it is resistant to many antibiotics. It can cause pneumonia, sepsis, and meningitis. It is spread person to person and is not airborne.
- ***Clostridium difficile***: Bacteria prevalent in people that have been on antibiotics. It can cause runny and uncontrolled diarrhea up to 20 times a day with severe abdominal cramping and can cause colitis. It is passed in feces and spread to surfaces and food when people who are infected don't wash their hands with soap and water. Antibacterial gel is not effective and does not work to stop contamination. It is not airborne.

## PRESSURE SORES/ULCERS

**Pressure sores/ulcers**, otherwise known as **decubitus ulcers**, are damage to the skin from being in one position for too long. The most common areas for pressure sores are over bony prominences such as the sacrum, ankles, back, elbows, and heels. People at greatest risk have mobility deficits causing difficulty in changing positions and likely spend the majority of their time in bed or in a chair or recliner. People with mobility deficits need to be frequently repositioned at a minimum of every 3 hours. **Repositioning** is the movement of the patient to relieve pressure either by themselves or with assistance from others. Terms such as **side lying** (lying on the left or right side with knees flexed and propped with pillows) or **floating** (can refer to the heels or buttock using pillows to offload pressure on the bony area) are often used in a hospital or skilled nursing setting. Air mattresses with alternating pressure is used to relieve pressure, and heel floating boots offload the heel pressure by suspending the heel over an open space to avoid pressure and shearing. Depending on the setting, use of these types of devices can fall to the discretion of nurses or therapists.

## EDEMA

**Edema** is the abnormal accumulation of fluid in the body causing swelling and increased size to the area. Edema can be caused from venous insufficiency, kidney disorders, medications, heart failure, and pregnancy. When the edema causes pitting, it is likely due to vascular issues or systemic concerns with the liver, heart, or kidney. Pitting edema is based on the ability of the edematous area to "bounce back" when pressure is applied. This is tested by the medical professional pressing with a finger into the area of edema and determining the depth of the indentation and the time it takes for the area to recover. The level of pitting is then determined by a numerical scale from 1 to 4. Edema is treated with medications such as Lasix, compression, and elevation of the affected area.

| Level | Depth | Time |
|-------|-------|------|
| 1 | 2 mm (not noticeable) | Immediately |
| 2 | 3–4 mm (minimal dent/depression) | <15 seconds |
| 3 | 5–6 mm (moderate dent/depression) | 10–30 seconds |
| 4 | 8 mm or greater (significant dent/depression) | >20 seconds |

## CONTRACTURES VS. SPASTICITY

A **contracture** is an often-permanent shortening or tightening of the muscles, tissues, or tendons creating a deformity (usually flexion) of a joint. Contractures can be orthopedic or neurological in causation. They can be skin based, muscular based, or joint based. They are seen most often in burn patients, post stroke, cerebral palsy, and muscular dystrophy. Occupational therapy treatments can focus on strengthening the muscles around the contracture, adaptive techniques and devices, PAMs, splinting, fine motor skills and dexterity activity, preventing further contractures, and increasing ROM. **Spasticity** is a neurological condition caused by damage to the brain and spinal cord causing muscle tightness and continuous contractions. It is often painful and can cause uncontrollable spasms of the upper and lower extremities. Treatment is the same as for contractures and is designed to reduce muscle tone. Patients with spasticity are often prescribed Botox injections and oral medications to assist with the therapy process.

## TYPES OF LYMPHEDEMA

Lymphedema is a blockage in the lymphatic system causing an abnormal accumulation and pooling of protein-rich lymph fluid. It can be primary or secondary. **Primary lymphedema** is due to a genetic condition causing issues with the lymphatic system. **Secondary lymphedema** is because of trauma, infection, or surgery with the most common cause being cancer treatment. There is no cure for lymphedema, but it can be managed with a course of treatment called **complete decongestive therapy (CDT)**. CDT is considered the best course of treatment and is the gold standard for lymphedema treatment. It is a combination of manual lymph drainage, skin and nail care, compression, and exercise. There are two phases of CDT: the intensive/decongestive phase and the self-management phase. In the decongestive phase, treatment is performed by a certified lymphedema therapist (CLT) and includes manual lymph drainage, bandaging, skin and nail care, and exercise. Once the size of the area has decreased, the self-management phase begins. This includes self-manual lymph drainage, self-bandaging and compression garments, skin and nail care, and exercise. This is a growing practice area for occupational therapy. To participate in certification, you must be an RN, OT/COTA, PT/PTA, MD/DO/DC, or an MT. A certification class of 135 hours and an exam will provide training to allow a therapist to be considered a CLT, and after a test through the Lymphology Association of North America, a therapist can use the CLT-LANA credential.

## ETIOLOGY OF BURNS

Burns can be thermal (flame, liquid, or steam), chemical (acids or bases, industrial/work accidents), or electrical (voltage). The initial treatment of the burn unit is stabilizing the patient, managing pain, and preventing infection. Burns are classified by the level of tissue that is involved and the amount of surface area affected. There are five categories for depth of burn injuries:

- **Superficial** (first-degree): Like a sunburn. Dry, red skin that is sore. Involves the epidermis only. Heals in 5 to 7 days with no scars and benefits from lotion and cream.
- **Superficial partial-thickness** (second-degree): Blanches with pressure, blisters that weep, moderate edema and fluid drainage, painful because it involves the epidermis and papillary dermis. Heals in 12 to 14 days with minimal scarring.
- **Deep partial-thickness** (second-degree): Mottled skin, sensation is altered, blanches to pressure. Light touch impaired, but deep pressure is intact. Involves the epidermis and dermis. May require surgical intervention. Significant scars and pigment damage to the skin.
- **Full-thickness** (third-degree): Mottled skin, no ability to sense pain, temperature, or pressure. Dry and rigid wounds. Involves the epidermis, dermis, and subcutaneous tissues. Will need surgery to close wounds and for grafting. Significant scarring and potential for contractures.
- **Subdermal**: The skin looks dry and charred. Deep tissues, muscles, and tendons are exposed. Involves the epidermis and dermis and destroys the subcutaneous tissue. Will need surgery and possible amputation of limbs. Significant scars and contractures are likely.

## RULE OF NINES

The rule of nines is a formula used to determine the percentage of the body that is affected by burns. Each body part is assigned a value that is a multiple of 9%. This is the easiest way to determine the burn size and guide treatment for the physician. The role of the OT in the burn unit can vary based on the severity of the burn. OTs can provide early mobility, positioning, ROM, splinting, edema management, and ADL training with adaptive equipment. Often, there will be concurrent treatments with physical therapy initially in the burn unit for patient activity tolerance and for the safety of the patient. Pain is a significant barrier to participation, and you may only get one shot to get a patient up and moving and readjusted in bed. Important areas to include in the evaluation that are burn-unit-specific include the total body surface area with the location of the burn, joints impacted with detailed ROM of that joint, the degree/level of the burn, if there is an inhalation injury, the types of dressings used and a schedule of when they are changed, and medications needed for pain and pressor drugs and when they are given.

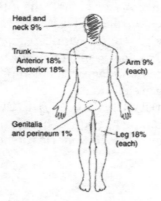

## SKIN GRAFTS AND SKIN FLAPS

A **skin graft** is a surgical procedure in which skin is taken from one place on the body and moved to another location to replace damaged skin. Cadaver skin and pig skin can also be used as a temporary cover. Skin grafts can be split-thickness or full-thickness. A split-thickness graft is when the graft includes the epidermis and some of the dermis and usually comes from the buttocks, back, abdomen, and outer thigh. A full-thickness graft includes removing all of the epidermis and dermis, and this is more delicate for smaller grafts coming from the clavicle, forearm, abdomen, and groin. Postsurgical placement of the graft, the patient should be on bedrest with no ROM on any joints that the graft crosses for five days. Often a wound VAC will be in place to promote skin graft adherence and healing. This will also help to prevent shearing of the graft when the patient is ambulating and moving. A **skin flap** is healthy skin and tissue including its own vascular supply that is moved from a donor site over the affected damaged area. A flap is used to cover a deeper, more complex wound. Therapy is guided by physician protocols, but patients are generally on bedrest for 7 to 14 days and then begin a postoperative dangling protocol in which the patient sits on the edge of the bed (EOB) supported and lets the LE hang off the EOB, slowly increasing the time from 5 minutes based on tolerance.

## WOUND CARE THERAPY

Many of the patients you see in your practice will have wounds in addition to the reason you are seeing them. This can have a significant impact on functional abilities. To become a certified wound care professional, you must be an LPN/RN/NP, PA, PT/PTA, OT/COTA, MD, or DO. **Wound care therapy** is provided by PTs and OTs with additional training and certification, and it is most often in an outpatient setting. Treatment can last from weeks to in some cases years depending on the type of wounds and the rate of healing. Wound care therapists are unique because they address wound healing, but they often provide interventions to support healing using mobility and positioning as needed. Treatment sessions include the following:

- measurement and documentation of the wound
- cleaning of the wound
- debridement
- modalities such as e-stim or mist therapy
- wound dressing
- education to the patient, caregivers, and the family on wound care and dressing changes

## STAGES OF WOUND HEALING

There are four stages of wound healing that overlap as healing progresses. These are the hemostasis, inflammation, proliferation, and maturation phases. When grouped together, the process can be called the inflammatory process. When a wound first occurs, the blood clots and forms a barrier to stop the bleeding and forms a scab. This is called **hemostasis.** The goal of the **inflammation phase** is to destroy bacteria and remove debris to encourage new tissue growth. The **proliferative phase** closes and fills the wound with connective tissue and new blood vessels until the wound is completely covered. In the **maturation phase**, the new tissue becomes more flexible and stronger. This process can continue for up to 2 years once the wound is closed.

## WOUND DEBRIDEMENT

**Surgical debridement** is performed only by a physician and is the removal of live and necrotic tissue. **Wound debridement** is the removal of dead and unhealthy tissue to promote healing and tissue regeneration by a professional with wound care certification using a scalpel, scissors, forceps, or tweezers. The scope of practice and regulations can vary between states. Patients are encouraged to eat diets high in protein because this helps to repair damaged tissue and promote new tissue growth. Patients are encouraged to stop smoking because smoking causes the arteries to become narrow, decreasing blood flow to the skin, which will slow wound healing. Patients are encouraged to keep pressure off the wound; to elevate the affected area to decrease edema; and to avoid swimming, hot tubs, and baths because they can cause the wound to become infected.

## WOUND STAGING IN PRESSURE ULCERS

**Wound staging** is a numerical scale used to classify wounds based on the depth of the wound and soft-tissue damage. Wounds can be grouped into four classifications or can be deemed unstageable.

| Classification | Descriptor |
| --- | --- |
| Stage I | Nonblanching and intact skin. Difference in color, temperature, and edema. |
| Stage II | Superficial ulcer that can present as a blister or indentation on the skin. Affects the epidermis and dermis and may have minimal drainage. |
| Stage III | Deep ulcer that looks like a deep indentation or crater. Moves to the subcutaneous layer and may have necrotic damage and some drainage. |
| Stage IV | May be deep enough to reach the bone and muscle. Highly necrotic with significant drainage. May have tracts and tunneling. |
| Unstageable | Ulcers covered with slough (dead and necrotic tissue that is yellow) or eschar (dead and necrotic tissue that is black). |

## TREATMENT MODALITIES USED IN WOUND CARE

There are multiple options used to treat wounds and promote wound healing. These are used as adjunct treatments that may help shorten the length of treatment and reduce pain and inflammation.

- **Hyperbaric oxygen therapy**: Increasing oxygen helps in wound healing. This therapy exposes the wound area to 100% oxygen at a pressure that is greater than normal through a boot or chamber to isolate the area.
- **Electrical stimulation (e-stim)**: Increases healing by increasing capillary density and improving the wound oxygenation, which encourages granulation. This is done by placing electrode pads around the wound and using a conducting agent to stimulate growth.
- **Pulsed lavage**: This is a type of hydrotherapy. It uses a pressurized saline solution to irrigate and debride wounds of necrotic tissue.
- **Whirlpool**: This is a type of hydrotherapy. It submerges the area in water and removes debris and surface bacteria. It also helps remove bandaging that has adhered to the wound. It works to remove significant amounts of necrotic tissue. *mechanical*
- **Compression therapy**: Compression works by increasing blood flow activity by strengthening vein support improving circulation and decreasing edema. Compression can be in the form of bandages or garments.
- **Negative pressure vacuum therapy**: A vacuum dressing is applied to promote wound healing. A sealed wound dressing attached to a pump creates negative pressure in the wound. This brings the wound edges together, removes infection, and actively encourages granulation.
- **Ultrasound mist therapy**: This is a low-frequency ultrasound with a saline mist that allows for wound cleaning and debridement and removal of slough and bacteria.

## TYPES OF SCARRING

A scar is a mark that is left on the skin after an injury or abrasion has fully healed. There are four categories of scars: atrophic, hypertrophic, keloid, and contracture.

| Type of Scar | Description |
| --- | --- |
| Atrophic scars | Sunken or dented-in appearance, common acne scars. The skin was unable to create collagen to fill and close the area. They are caused by chicken pox, acne, and staph infections. |
| Hypertrophic scars | Red, hard, and raised. The skin produced too much collagen during the healing process. They are caused by surgical incision, acne, burns, and chicken pox. |
| Keloid scars | Lumpy, elevated, larger than the original injury site, and dark in color. The skin produced too much collagen during the healing process. They are often caused by acne or surgical incisions. |
| Contracture scars | Most often seen in burn patients. Increased production of collagen causes attachments to structures that will limit mobility. |

## SCAR MASSAGE

**Scar massage** is a technique used to release and mobilize the adhesions between the dermis and deeper internal structures such as fascia, muscles, tendons, and sometimes organs. When the dermis is compromised by injury or surgery, it forms new collagen fibers that attach to the underlying structures to close the wound and repair itself. Scar massage can help prevent tissue buildup and puckering at the scar site, which can cause decreased mobility and may compromise ROM. Scar massage should only begin when the wound is fully healed and any scabs have fallen off in the healing process. Scar massage begins with the application of heat in order to warm the tissue and increase circulation. Depending on the placement of the scar, moist heat or paraffin can be used. When the area has been warmed and dried, lotion is used as a moisturizer and lubricant so the massage can be performed without painful friction. Placing your index and middle fingers along the ridge that is felt under the scar, make small, firm circles along the length of the scar. Moderate pressure is used to reduce swelling in the scar and break up the underlying tightness and adhesions. Family members or the patient themselves can be taught this technique as part of their home exercise program (HEP), and it should be performed 5 to 10 minutes three times a day until the incision feels like the normal skin around the scar.

## RETROGRADE MASSAGE

Swelling and edema are a common occurrence after injury or surgery. They are caused by an increase in the interstitial fluid volume. **Retrograde massage** is a common technique used by OTs in all settings to address and reduce swelling. The massage consists of manually moving fluid distal to proximal from the tips of the fingers back toward the heart so that it can be reabsorbed into the bloodstream. Aggressive management of edema is important to reduce pain, reduce joint stiffness, and increase mobility and function for ADLs. Elevation is the important first step to reduce edema in your patient, and it can be quite successful when combined with exercise. Contraindications of retrograde massage include the following:

- Deep vein thrombosis (DVT): If the swelling is caused by a clot, massage could cause the clot to dislodge and be sent to the lungs.
- Heart conditions (congestive heart failure, high blood pressure): The patient's heart may not be able to manage the amount of fluid being pushed back toward it during the massage.
- Cellulitis: This is a bacterial skin infection that can cause a patient to become septic if the infection spreads into the circulatory system.

- Active cancer: Some cancers can spread lymphatically, and massage increases the circulation of lymph. (The patient's physician will determine if massage can be part of the treatment plan.)

## THERAPEUTIC TAPING

Therapeutic taping is more commonly known as Kinesio Taping, which is a brand of therapy tape that has become the mainstream lexicon. There are dozens of brands of tape on the market including RockTape, Kinesio Tape, and SpiderTech. The goal of therapy tape is to provide support to muscles and joints without limiting ROM, and it can also improve circulation, decrease pain, and reposition and support a joint subluxation. Tape can be used to inhibit a muscle pattern or spasm to decrease pain, or it can facilitate muscle movement for increased muscle tone and contraction patterns. The use of tape needs to be documented well on the POC if it will be used in treatment.

## PAMs

According to AOTA's Occupational Therapy Practice Act, **physical agent modalities (PAMs)** are "techniques that produce a response in soft tissue through the use of light, water, temperature, sound, or electricity." They are modalities that enhance treatment by decreasing pain, stiffness, and spasm. PAMs can be separated into three categories: superficial thermal agents, deep thermal agents, and electrotherapeutic agents/mechanical devices. When a modality is combined with therapeutic exercise or manual therapy techniques, outcomes improve significantly. The contraindications for PAMs are active cancer, pacemaker, and pregnancy and cognitive, sensory, and vascular impairments. The ability to use PAMs varies on a state-to-state basis with some requiring additional certification to use them in treatment. The AOTA website has links to each state's rules and regulations.

### CATEGORIES OF PAMs

The following are the three categories of physical agent modalities:

- **Superficial thermal** agents are used to create temperature changes that will promote blood flow and healing. They only impact above the subcutaneous fat layer, which insulates the deeper tissues and bone from the effects. Superficial agents are hot and cold packs, fluidotherapy, hydrotherapy/whirlpool, infrared, and paraffin. Superficial modalities can penetrate 1–3 cm.
- **Deep thermal** agents affect the deep tissues, muscles and bone. They include: ultrasound, diathermy and phonophoresis.
- **Electrotherapeutic/Mechanical** PAMs use electricity to facilitate tissue healing, improve muscle strength and endurance, and decrease edema and pain. They include neuromuscular electrical stimulation (NMES), functional electrical stimulation (FES), transcutaneous electrical nerve stimulation (TENS), iontophoresis, continuous passive movement (CPM), and a sequential compression device (SCD)

### INDICATIONS, CONTRAINDICATIONS, AND APPROPRIATE CLINICAL APPLICATION OF VARIOUS PAMs

#### ULTRASOUND

**Effect**: Uses a high-frequency sound wave that can create thermal and nonthermal (tissue repair) effects. Tissue repair, increasing flexibility, decrease pain, muscle spasms, and swelling. It can penetrate 5 cm.

**Contraindication/Precautions**: Impaired sensation, blood clots, significant swelling, active cancers, infection, open wounds, cognitive impairments, metal implants, pregnancy, pacemakers, at a fracture site that is healing over bony prominences, or ischemic tissue over the eyes or gonads or over the spinal cord after laminectomy.

**Conditions/Applications**: Bursitis, frozen shoulder, myositis, soft-tissue injuries, and breaking down scar tissue.

## DIATHERMY

**Effect**: Uses high-frequency electromagnetic energy. Can be shortwave or microwave. Increases ROM and flexibility and decreases pain and swelling. It can penetrate 3 cm.

**Contraindication/Precautions**: Implantable electronic devices such as a pacemaker or spinal cord stimulator, malignant tumors, pregnancy, active tuberculosis, impaired sensation, blood clots, cognitive impairments, metal implants, and ischemic tissue over the eyes or gonads.

**Conditions/Applications**: Joint contractures or adhesions, muscle spasms, bursitis, and muscle sprains or strains.

## HEAT (MOIST HEAT, CONTRAST BATHS)

**Effect:** Heat increases blood flow, increases the inflammatory response, increases joint mobility and ROM, helps reabsorb hematomas, and is analgesic for the patient. Moist heat pads are kept in a hydrocollator in water at 170ºF. Six to eight layers of towels should be placed between the patient and the pad. It is conductive heat that penetrates 1/4 to 1/2 inch.

**Contraindication/Precautions:** Cardiac insufficiency, pregnancy, open wounds, acute inflammatory conditions, hemorrhage concerns or disorders, thrombophlebitis, peripheral vascular disease (PVD), deep vein thrombosis (DVT), active cancer, radiation treatment, blood or skin infections, cognitive deficits.

**Conditions/Applications:** Chronic inflammatory conditions, chronic pain chronic muscle spasm, joint contractures, and to address ROM deficits before manual therapy.

## COLD (ICE PACKS, CONTRAST BATH)

**Effect:** Cold reduces inflammation and edema by decreasing blood flow. Used to control acute pain and edema post injury; reduce inflammation; and decrease bruising, hemorrhage, and muscle spasm.

**Contraindication/Precautions:** Raynaud's disease history of syncope regenerating peripheral nerve, poor circulation, angina, open wounds, hypertension (HTN), and cognitive deficits.

**Conditions/Applications:** Acute injury and chronic pain. Postsurgical pain and edema. Acute or chronic muscle spasm

## HYDROTHERAPY/WHIRLPOOL

**Effect:** Cold whirlpool is 50°F to 65°F, and warm is 90°F to 110°F. Convection heat penetrates to 1/4 to 1/2 inch.

**Contraindication/Precautions:** Cardiac conditions, diabetic issues, hypertension, syncope, and cognitive deficits.

**Conditions/Applications:** Decreased ROM, chronic inflammatory conditions, burns, debridement.

## PHONOPHORESIS

**Effect**: Uses topical anti-inflammatory medications with ultrasound to increase tissue repair and flexibility and decrease pain and swelling. Can break down tissue based on the medication used. It can penetrate 10 cm.

**Contraindication/Precautions**: Acute inflammation, breast implant, healing fractures, growing epiphyseal plates, decreased sensation and decreased cognition. Implantable electronic devices such as a pacemaker or spinal cord stimulator, malignant tumors, pregnancy.

**Conditions/Applications**: Tendinitis, bursitis, tennis or golfer's elbow, osteoarthritis (OA), De Quervain syndrome, and carpal tunnel syndrome.

## TRANSCUTANEOUS ELECTRICAL NERVE STIMULATION (TENS)

**Effect**: Stimulates motor and sensory nerves to decrease pain.

**Contraindication/Precautions**: Pregnancy, epilepsy, over the carotid sinus, or over a pacemaker or spinal cord stimulator.

**Conditions/Applications**: Chronic pain, spinal radiculopathy.

## NEUROMUSCULAR ELECTRICAL STIMULATION (NMES)

**Effect**: This is a device that sends electric impulses to nerves in order to cause a muscle to contract. It helps increase strength and ROM and falls under the heading "neuromuscular reeducation."

**Contraindication/Precautions**: Hemorrhage concerns or disorders, DVT, active cancer, radiation treatment, blood or skin infections, cognitive deficits, neuropathy, active tuberculosis (TB), over the carotid sinus, over a pacemaker or spinal cord stimulator.

**Conditions/Applications**: Post stroke, cerebral palsy, TBI, spinal cord injury.

## FUNCTIONAL ELECTRICAL STIMULATION

**Effect**: A form of NMES used to stimulate a paralyzed muscle.

**Contraindication/Precautions**: Hemorrhage concerns or disorders, DVT, active cancer, radiation treatment, blood or skin infections, cognitive deficits, neuropathy, active TB, over the carotid sinus, over a pacemaker or spinal cord stimulator.

**Conditions/Applications**: Muscle atrophy, weakness and spasm.

## IONTOPHORESIS

**Effect**: Uses a direct current to move ions through the skin for pain management and wound healing.

**Contraindication/Precautions**: Broken skin, acute hemorrhage and acute injury.

**Conditions/Applications**: Reduces pain, inflammation, edema, and muscle spasms.

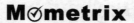

### CONTINUOUS PASSIVE MOVEMENT (CPM)

**Effect**: Most commonly seen after knee surgery but can also be for the hand. This machine allows passive flexion and extension of the joint post-surgery to prevent tightness and decrease edema and stiffness. It can be adjusted in speed and degree of flexion.

**Contraindication/Precautions**: Unstable fracture, ROM restrictions from surgery, DVT.

### SEQUENTIAL COMPRESSION DEVICE

**Effect**: Alternating compression devices that can be worn up to 18 hours a day. They are often seen in the hospital and post-surgery when a patient is not moving around and ambulating as normal in order to prevent blood clots.

**Contraindication/Precautions**: DVT, compartment syndrome, open wounds.

### PARAFFIN

**Effect**: The extremity is dipped in paraffin 6 to 8 times till a crust is formed and then wrapped in plastic immediately following the last dip to retain the heat. Paraffin baths should be maintained at temp of 126ºF It is conduction heat that penetrates to ¼ of an inch.

**Contraindication/Precautions**: Open wounds, rashes, acute episodes of inflammatory arthritis and cognitive deficits.

**Conditions/Applications**: Chronic inflammatory conditions, increasing ROM limitation after splinting or casting, softening the skin for scar massage work.

### INFRARED

**Effect**:  Electromagnetic radiation that penetrates the tissue to reduce pain reduce muscle spasm decrease inflammation wound and tissue repair. It is a superficial dry heat that penetrates up to 3cm.

**Contraindication/Precautions**: Cardiac insufficiency, pregnancy, open wounds, acute inflammatory conditions, hemorrhage concerns or disorders, thrombophlebitis, PVD, DVT, active cancer, radiation treatment, blood or skin infections, cognitive deficits.

**Conditions/Applications**: Arthritis, chronic pain, Neuropathy, Muscle strain, wound care, chronic ulcers and pain reduction.

### FLUIDOTHERAPY

**Effect**: This is a dry-heat modality that uses organic particles circulated by hot air. The affected area is placed in a machine in which it is warmed by circulating corn husks. The temperature is maintained at 110ºF to 125ºF. Heat increases blood flow, increases the inflammatory response, increases joint mobility and ROM, helps reabsorb hematomas, and is analgesic for the patient. It is convection heat that penetrates to 1/4 inch.

**Contraindication/Precautions**: Open wounds, rashes, acute episodes of inflammatory arthritis, and cognitive deficits.

**Conditions/Applications**: Desensitize after nerve injury or surgery, chronic inflammatory conditions, chronic pain, chronic muscle spasm, joint contractures, and to address ROM deficits before manual therapy.

## SCI

A **spinal cord injury (SCI)** is caused by damage to the spinal cord and or nerve roots. SCIs are permanent. SCIs can be complete or incomplete. In an incomplete injury, there is some sensation that is still intact below the level of the injury. In a complete injury, there is no sensory or motor movement below the level of the injury. Quadriplegia/Tetraplegia is an injury at the level of the cervical vertebrae, and there is no movement of the upper or lower limbs. This is the most serious because it can also impact breathing, bowels, and sexual function. Paraplegia is an injury at the thoracic or lumbar vertebral regions that impacts the lower extremities but not the upper extremities.

| Effect on Occupational Performance | Therapeutic Treatment |
|---|---|
| Depends on the level of injury. All areas of ADLs and IADLs including bowel, bladder, sexual function, respiratory function, mobility and motor skills, vision, swallowing, speech, and leisure activity. | Home evaluation, weight-bearing, ROM, transfer training, posture and seating interventions, skin care, caregiver training, adaptive techniques for self-care, eating and feeding techniques, fatigue management, energy conservation, home exercise program, aggressive fine and gross motor strengthening, modalities, coordination and dexterity activity, cognition, and sequencing. |

## ARTHRITIS

Arthritis is inflammation of the joints. It is considered a rheumatic disease, which means that it can affect your joints, tendons, ligaments, bones, and muscles. The two most common types of arthritis are osteoarthritis (OA) and rheumatoid arthritis (RA).

### EFFECT OF OA ON OCCUPATIONAL PERFORMANCE

**Osteoarthritis (OA)** is a degenerative joint disease. It is not a systemic disease. It is due to normal wear and tear on the joints, injury, and being overweight. There may be crepitus (audible and palpable "crunching" in the joint) and morning stiffness in the joints and stiffness after sitting or inactivity. There is no cure.

| Effect on Occupational Performance | Therapeutic Treatment |
|---|---|
| Can affect all areas of ADLs and IADLs depending on severity. Difficulty using adaptive equipment such as gripping a walker or cane and donning compression garments. | Physical agent modalities (PAMs), for example, heat or cold, to assist with pain management, limb elevation, compression garments, exercise, and splinting for inflammation and edema. Education in joint protection and energy conservation techniques and adaptive equipment. |

## EFFECT OF RA ON OCCUPATIONAL PERFORMANCE

**Rheumatoid Arthritis (RA)** is a chronic disease that causes inflammation of the synovium of the joint and is most often seen in the hands and feet. It is unique in that it presents equally on both sides of the body. There is no cure.

| Effect on Occupational Performance | Therapeutic Treatment |
|---|---|
| Can affect all areas of ADLs and IADLs depending on severity. Difficulty using adaptive equipment such as gripping a walker or cane and donning compression garments. | Electrostimulation (e-stim) for pain management. Cold/heat modalities with cold in acute stages and hot in chronic stages. Joint protection strategies, splinting, compression, exercise, education in joint protection and energy conservation techniques, and adaptive equipment. |

## FIBROMYALGIA

**Fibromyalgia** is a chronic condition of overall body pain/widespread pain, sleep disturbances, stress, and fatigue. It is difficult to diagnosis because it is usually seen in conjunction with other disorders such as chronic fatigue syndrome, irritable bowel syndrome, anxiety, and depression. The cause is unknown, but symptoms can often be treated with medications and reductions in stress.

| Effect on Occupational Performance | Therapeutic Treatment |
|---|---|
| Can affect all areas of ADLs and IADLs depending on severity. Mobility and fine and gross motor skills are impaired. | There is no overall consensus on the treatment of choice. Stretching programs exist, although many patients complain that exercise can cause increased pain. E-stim can help localized pain symptoms, adaptive techniques, energy conservation, pain management, relaxation techniques, problem solving, and sleep hygiene. |

## PARKINSON'S DISEASE

**Parkinson's disease** is a degenerative disorder of the central nervous system. It is a progressive disease, and there is not yet a cure. It is caused when the neurons in the brain that produce dopamine stop working. Symptoms are **bradykinesia** (slow movement and difficulty moving the body the way it is intended to move), **hypokinesia** (partial or complete loss of muscle movement), rigidity, and resting tremors.

| Effect on Occupational Performance | Therapeutic Treatment |
|---|---|
| Will impact all areas of ADLs and IADLs. Mobility and motor skills are impaired. Cognition, problem solving, swallowing, speech, and leisure activity are affected. | Home safety evaluations to optimize environment, bed mobility, transfer training, posture and seating interventions, caregiver training, adaptive techniques for self-care, eating and feeding techniques, fatigue management, visual or rhythmic cues for mobility, handwriting interventions, BIG and LOUD programs. Lee Silverman Voice Treatment (LSVT) BIG is an exercise program, and LSVT LOUD is a speech program designed to use large movement and loud vocalization activity that can be carried over to daily life for improved function. |

## MS

***Multiple sclerosis (MS)*** is an abnormal response of the body's immune system affecting the central nervous system that damages the myelin sheath around the nerve fibers. Symptoms include pain, vertigo, gait issues, involuntary movement, muscle rigidity, overactive reflexes, muscle cramping, and tremors.

| Effect on Occupational Performance | Therapeutic Treatment |
| --- | --- |
| All areas of ADLs and IADLs. Mobility and motor skills are impaired. Cognition, problem solving, swallowing, speech, and leisure activity are affected. | Home safety evaluations to optimize environment, bed mobility, transfer training, posture and seating interventions, caregiver training, adaptive techniques for self-care, eating and feeding techniques, fatigue management, home exercise program, fine and gross motor skill strengthening, energy conservation, coordination and dexterity activity, cognitive training, and compensatory strategies. |

## ALS/LOU GEHRIG'S DISEASE

**Amyotrophic lateral sclerosis (ALS)/Lou Gehrig's disease** is a motor neuron disease in which nerve cells gradually break down and die. It affects control of the muscles compromising the ability to talk, swallow, walk, and breathe. ALS is always fatal, usually within 3–5 years of diagnosis. The most common cause of death is respiratory failure:

| Effect on Occupational Performance | Therapeutic Treatment |
| --- | --- |
| All areas of ADLs and IADLs. Mobility and motor skills are impaired. Swallowing, speech, and leisure activity are affected. | Home safety evaluations to optimize environment, bed mobility, transfer training, posture and seating interventions, caregiver training, adaptive techniques for self-care, eating and feeding techniques, fatigue management, energy conservation, home exercise program, fine and gross motor skill strengthening, coordination and dexterity activity, cognitive training, and compensatory strategies. Alternative methods of communication/assistive technology and text-to-speech devices are used. |

## GBS

**Guillain-Barré syndrome (GBS)** is a rare neurological autoimmune disorder characterized by rapid-onset muscle weakness caused by the immune system damaging the peripheral nervous system. The immune system attacks healthy nerves usually after a respiratory or gastrointestinal (GI) infection. People will recover from GBS but will often have residual muscle weakness.

| Effect on Occupational Performance | Therapeutic Treatment |
| --- | --- |
| All areas of ADLs and IADLs. Mobility and motor skills are impaired. Swallowing, speech, and leisure activity are affected. There are toileting issues and sensory issues in the hands and feet. | Bed mobility, home evaluation, transfer training, posture and seating interventions, caregiver training, adaptive techniques for self-care, eating and feeding techniques, fatigue management, energy conservation, home exercise program, aggressive fine and gross motor skill strengthening, and coordination and dexterity activities. |

## CVA

A **cerebrovascular accident (CVA)** is the term used for a stroke. The blood flow to the brain is stopped by a blockage or from a rupture of a vessel causing a lack of oxygen to the brain and the death of cells. There are two types of stroke: **ischemic and hemorrhagic.** An ischemic stroke is caused by a blockage, and a hemorrhagic stroke is caused by the rupture of a blood vessel. An ischemic stroke can be embolic (when a clot is formed and travels to the brain lodging there and causing damage) or thrombotic (when a clot is formed inside the brain).

| Effect on Occupational Performance | Therapeutic Treatment |
|---|---|
| Depends on severity. All areas of ADLs and IADLs, mobility and motor skills swallowing, speech, and leisure activity can be compromised. | Home evaluation, weight-bearing, range of motion (ROM), transfer training, posture and seating interventions, caregiver training, adaptive techniques for self-care, eating and feeding techniques, fatigue management, energy conservation, home exercise programs, aggressive fine and gross motor skill strengthening, coordination and dexterity activities, cognition, sequencing, and impulse control. |

## TBI

**Traumatic brain injury (TBI)** is usually from an acute injury or trauma to the head in which brain tissue has likely been damaged and is usually seen in falls, combat accidents, automobile/motorcycle accidents, seizures, sports injuries, or violence. The effects can be permanent. TBIs can be classified as mild or severe. Mild identifies a loss of consciousness of less than 30 minutes. Often this is followed by confusion, mood swings, headaches, memory issues, difficulty with attention to task, and frustration causing the person to be quick to anger. In a severe TBI, loss of consciousness is for more than 30 minutes and there is usually an acute penetration injury of the skull/brain. Patients can often be in a coma for a time, and they will have significant cognitive and mood changes, deficits in gross and fine motor skills, speech and sensory issues, as well as vision issues. Some deficits may be permanent, and rehabilitation will be ongoing for years.

| Effect on Occupational Performance | Therapeutic Treatment |
|---|---|
| Depends on severity. All areas of ADLs and IADLs, mobility and motor skills, vision, swallowing, speech, and leisure activity can be compromised. | Home evaluation, weight-bearing, ROM, transfer training, posture and seating interventions, caregiver training, adaptive techniques for self-care, eating and feeding techniques, fatigue management, energy conservation, home exercise program, aggressive fine and gross motor skill strengthening, coordination and dexterity activities, cognition, sequencing, and impulse control. |

## DSM-5

The **Diagnostic and Statistical Manual of Mental Disorders, Fifth Edition (DSM-5)** is a book published by the American Psychiatric Association that is used to diagnose mental disorders. The diagnoses in the book are depression and depressive disorders. The most recent revision was in 2013. The manual describes symptoms, statistics about each diagnosis, effects of treatment, and treatment approaches. As OTs, we look at the disorders in this book and treat the psychosocial symptoms. Occupational therapy found its beginnings in mental health in the early 1900s working with soldiers injured in war, and it was craft and activity oriented. These days, OTs work with independence with ADLs, coping skills, leisure and work skills, social participation and promoting overall wellness, life satisfaction and quality of life. Goals can address self-esteem and acceptance, relationships both personal and in the workplace, orientation to reality, goal-directed activities, and self-awareness identifying triggers that lead to unwanted behaviors.

## DIAGNOSIS OF SCHIZOPHRENIA

**Schizophrenia** is a chemical imbalance in the brain that can cause thoughts and behaviors that seem out of touch from reality. It may cause hallucinations and delusions, including hearing voices.

| Effect on occupational performance | Therapeutic treatment |
| --- | --- |
| All aspects of life are affected: work, socialization, ADLs, productivity, cognition, processing and decision making, self-awareness, decision making, motivation, judgment, and safety. | Self-care, including medication management, personal hygiene, and ADLs and functional skills such as meal preparation and money management. Leisure exploration, productivity focus/skills for job search, coordination and body awareness, regulating arousal and alertness, decision making, time management, coping skills with adaptive strategies, group activities for socialization, and outings into the community for practicing appropriate behaviors and social skills. |

## DIAGNOSIS OF SUBSTANCE ABUSE

**Substance abuse** is dependence and overuse of an addictive substance to the point that it has a negative impact on a person's life. Generally, this involves alcohol and drugs.

| Effect on occupational performance | Therapeutic treatment |
| --- | --- |
| All aspects of life are affected: work, socialization, ADLs, productivity, cognition, processing and decision making, self-awareness, decision making, motivation, judgment, and safety. | Coping skills, understanding negative consequences, adaptive techniques, social interactions and parenting skills, relaxation techniques, self-care and ADLs, decision making, and leisure exploration. |

## DIAGNOSIS OF OBSESSIVE-COMPULSIVE DISORDER

**Obsessive-compulsive disorder** is an excessive, unhealthy preoccupation or obsession with order, cleanliness, control, and perfectionism.

| Effect on occupational performance | Therapeutic treatment |
| --- | --- |
| All aspects of life are affected: work, socialization, ADLs, productivity, cognition, processing and decision making, self-awareness, decision making, motivation, coping skills, concept formation, judgment, and safety. | Work therapy; stress management; self-care, including medication management, personal hygiene, and ADLs; functional skills such as meal preparation; sensory activities; leisure skills; time management; functional activities and crafts; coping skills; regulating arousal and alertness; and decision making. |

## DIAGNOSIS OF BIPOLAR DISORDER

**Bipolar disorder** is a chemical imbalance in the brain that can cause mood swings from mania to depression with occasional suicidal thoughts or ideation.

| Effect on occupational performance | Therapeutic treatment |
|---|---|
| All aspects of life are affected: work, social, ADLs, productivity, cognition, processing and decision making, self-awareness, decision making, motivation, judgment, and safety. | Self-care, including medication management, personal hygiene, and ADLs and functional skills such as meal preparation and money management. Leisure exploration, productivity, coping skills, regulating arousal and alertness, decision making, identifying triggers, and establishing healthy routines and habits. |

## DIAGNOSIS OF BORDERLINE PERSONALITY DISORDER

**Borderline personality disorder** causes emotional instability and impulsivity affecting how you feel about yourself and others. It often causes feelings of worthlessness and insecurity.

| Effect on occupational performance | Therapeutic treatment |
|---|---|
| All aspects of life are affected: work, socialization, ADLs, productivity, cognition, processing and decision making, self-awareness, decision making, motivation, judgment, and safety. | Self-care, including medication management, personal hygiene and ADLs, functional skills such as meal preparation, and money management. Leisure exploration, productivity focus, coping skills, regulating arousal and alertness, decision making, time management, adaptive strategies, group activities for socialization, and outings into the community for practicing appropriate behaviors and social skills. |

## DIAGNOSIS OF POST-TRAUMATIC STRESS DISORDER

**Post-traumatic stress disorder** is a psychiatric disorder that can occur after participating in or witnessing a life-threatening event such as military service, accidents, traumatic events such as assault, and natural disasters.

| Effect on occupational performance | Therapeutic treatment |
|---|---|
| All aspects of life are affected: work, socialization, ADLs, productivity, cognition, processing and decision making, self-awareness, decision making, motivation, judgment, and safety. | Coping skills including identifying trauma triggers and environmental barriers, work- and social-based strategies, dissociation techniques, sensory diet. Self-care, including medication management, personal hygiene, and ADLs. Functional skills such as meal preparation and money management. Leisure exploration and productivity. |

## DIAGNOSIS OF ANXIETY

**Anxiety** is fear, stress, and worry to the point that it can interfere with daily life.

| Effect on occupational performance | Therapeutic treatment |
|---|---|
| All aspects of life are affected: work, socialization, ADLs, productivity, cognition, processing and decision making, self-awareness, decision making, motivation, judgment, and safety. | Stress relief, coping skills, meditation and relaxation techniques, self-care routine, home management, leisure and hobby exploration, decision making and problem solving, self-confidence, interpersonal skills, cognitive activities, and one-on-one and group activities. |

## DIAGNOSIS OF DEPRESSION

**Depression** is a persistent feeling of sadness, hopelessness, and worthlessness including loss of interest, isolation, and suicidal ideation.

| Effect on occupational performance | Therapeutic treatment |
|---|---|
| All aspects of life are affected: work, socialization, ADLs, productivity, cognition, processing and decision making, self-awareness, decision making, motivation, judgment, and safety. | Self-care routine, home management, leisure and hobby exploration, decision making and problem solving, self-confidence, stress relief and coping skills, self-expression, and interpersonal skills including socialization activities. |

## TYPES OF PLAY INTERVENTIONS/GAMES USED WITH A CHILD
### USED WITH A CHILD TO WORK ON CROSSING MIDLINE

**Crossing midline** is the ability to use your hands and legs to reach across your body. Crossing midline leads to **bilateral coordination**, which is the ability to use both sides of the body at the same time in organized, smooth, and controlled movement. The ability to cross midline impacts activities such as reading, writing, using utensils, throwing and catching, and visually scanning the environment. The following are interventions used to facilitate crossing midline:

- using a vertical surface such as a whiteboard to draw a large figure 8 on its side: ∞
- play catch or hit a balloon having the therapist change the angle that the ball is thrown to promote crossing midline
- sitting back to back and passing a ball back and forth around the side to each other
- dealing cards to multiple players
- seated marching touching the opposite hand to the knee that is raised
- playing Twister, beanbag toss, Simon Says
- playing balloon volley with a pool noodle held like a baseball bat
- play clapping games
- painting
- obstacle courses
- using vertical surfaces for activities (felt boards, magnet boards, card sorting, drawing).

### USED WITH A CHILD TO WORK ON UE MOBILITY/STRENGTH

UE mobility and strength are tied to trunk and core strength and have a direct impact on fine motor skills in a child. Strong trunk strength allows for movement of the arms and legs without extra support and provides stability to the shoulder girdle, spine, and pelvis. The following are interventions used to facilitate UE and core strength:

- wheelbarrow walking (therapist holds the child's feet, and the child walks on their hands)
- using a scooter board in prone
- playing board games, puzzles, coloring in prone on the floor
- playing board games and reaching activities in side lying
- animal walks
- tug of war
- activities in quadruped
- obstacle courses
- push-pull activities
- prone tasks such as life-size puzzles and coloring over an exercise or peanut ball.

## USED WITH A CHILD TO WORK ON MOBILITY/WEIGHT SHIFTING

Weight shifting is the ability to move the body's center of mass from one foot to the other without moving the feet. It is the foundation of postural control, body awareness in space, and stability. Weight shifting is a precursor to functional ambulation for all standing ADLs.

- use games on the Wii
- hula hoop
- wobble boards
- sitting on therapy balls, peanut balls, bolster, or wobble cushions while completing tasks
- tasks and games in high kneeling and quadruped (puzzles coloring, sorting, board games)
- swinging
- teeter totter
- Twister
- playing catch or balloon volley
- obstacle courses.

## USED WITH A CHILD TO WORK ON FINE MOTOR CONTROL AND HAND WRITING

Fine motor skills are based on the ability and the coordination of the small muscles in the hand to work together to create small, detailed and intricate movement. It is the fine motor ability that allows us to reach, grasp, write, manipulate, and move objects. Activities that can help encourage fine motor skills and handwriting include:

- using PlayDoh and TheraPutty to make shapes, letters, snip with scissors, manipulate and remove small beads of coins imbedded in it
- making paper clip chains or rubber band balls
- lacing and stringing beads
- playing with pop beads
- coloring, drawing, tracing, cutting, tearing paper, and using hole punches and stickers
- flicking beans across a surface by isolating each finger
- tweezer and clothespin activities
- attaching screws and bolts.

## USED WITH A CHILD TO WORK ON SENSORY PROCESSING

**Sensory integration activities** are a way to get kids to tolerate, process, and interpret the sensory input that they receive throughout the day. Once the area of concern has been determined, we can create tasks to help them regulate and process this input more effectively. The following activities can encourage sensory processing skills:

| Activity | Examples |
|---|---|
| Messy play | Hiding items in and playing with shaving cream, PlayDoh, slime, Gak, Funny Foam, Flubber, dirt, sand, and kinetic sand. |
| Heavy work | Using weighted blankets and lap pads, jumping, bouncing on balls, rocking, pushing, pulling, swinging, and being compressed or "squished." |
| Vibrating tools | Vibrating toothbrushes, massagers, chairs, and mats. |
| Aromatherapy | Using scent to relax or calm behaviors or drown out smells. You can use oils, candles, or a diffuser. |
| Vestibular activity | Trampolines, swings, scooter boards, teeter totters, and therapy balls. |

## USED WITH A CHILD TO WORK ON SOCIAL INTERACTION

Social skills are needed in order to have positive interactions and communicate with others on a daily basis and to participate actively as a functional member of society. Social skills help us determine what behavior is appropriate in social settings and include both verbal and nonverbal communication skills. You will most often work on social skills with children diagnosed with an autism spectrum disorder or Asperger's. The following are common intervention skills to work on social interactions:

- turn-taking games
- role-playing games
- watch-and-comment activities (watch an interaction and have the patient describe what they see and if it was appropriate)
- imitate games such as Simon Says
- emotion games (looking at pictures in a magazine and reporting if the person looks sad or happy/drawing an emotion out of a box and acting it out).

## USED WITH A CHILD TO WORK ON ADLS

Activities of daily living (ADLs) encompass all the activities that make up the tasks in your daily life, including things such as brushing teeth, buttoning and fastening clothes, toileting, eating, and using utensils. Using practical approaches for these skills is the easiest way to do this with a child and can include the following:

- having a tea party with real food to work on using utensils and cups
- making a recipe in the kitchen
- playing dress-up with clothes that have multiple fasteners
- tying shoes
- brushing their own teeth or brushing their toy's teeth
- cleaning up the therapy room.

## TYPES OF INTERVENTIONS USED TO ENCOURAGE SENSORY AROUSAL

Arousal is our level of alertness, and it determines how able we are to pay attention and respond appropriately to what is going on in our environment. Each person responds differently to a sensory event. Our sensory arousal is the level of input needed to detect and respond to sensory information. The following are activities that can increase and decrease sensory arousal:

- **Improve/Increase Arousal and Alertness**
  o Loud rhythmic music (listening and playing)
  o Bright light
  o Bright colors
  o Gross motor movement (jumping, spinning, running, sliding, scooter board)
  o Eating food with crunchy textures
  o Messy play
  o Parachute play and catch-and-release games
- **Decrease Arousal and Alertness**
  o Slow music
  o Warm drinks and food
  o Weighted vests, blankets
  o Slow rhythmic movement (swings or bouncing)
  o Heavy work (pushing and pulling)
  o Low light levels
  o Warm colors
  o Deep pressure/massage
  o Slow, repetitive movement activity

## TYPES OF INTERVENTIONS USED TO ENCOURAGE VISUAL MOTOR SKILLS

**Visual motor skills** involve the ability of the hands and eyes to work together to create an organized and coordinated movement. Use the following tasks:

| Activity | Skills |
|---|---|
| Dot pictures and grid pictures | address spatial perception, visual discrimination, and attention to detail. |
| Figure ground pictures | teach how to filter visual information that is not important so the patient can focus on the relevant visual information. |
| Mazes and dot-to-dot handouts | address spatial perception and visual discrimination; teach following horizontal, vertical, and diagonal lines. |
| Complete-the-picture games | involves understanding that letters, words, and numbers remain the same despite context and environment. |
| Cutting shapes and pictures | addresses fine motor coordination, bilateral coordination, and eye-hand coordination. |
| Lacing and threading | visual scanning, bilateral integration, motor planning. |
| Origami | bilateral integration, motor planning, visual discrimination, fine motor skills. |
| Playing catch | bilateral integration, bilateral coordination, and motor planning. |
| Geo boards | address spatial perception, visual discrimination, and attention to detail. |

## TYPES OF INTERVENTIONS USED TO ENCOURAGE COGNITIVE SKILLS

**Cognitive skills** are what makes everyday activity possible. Cognition helps us think and process, read and understand what we are reading, learn new concepts, remember, reason, and focus on tasks. These skills can be encouraged with the following tasks:

| Activity | Skills |
|---|---|
| **Multiple-choice (this-or-that)** | reasoning, grouping skills, inference skills, decision making, executive functioning, planning, and organizing |
| **Remembering and matching games** | focus, concentration, improving recall, and problem solving |
| **Sorting and classifying games** | grouping, labeling, recall, decision making, reasoning, and planning |
| **Imaginary play/acting out scenarios.** | safety awareness, decision making, appropriate behavior, focus, executive functioning, planning and organizing, and impulse control |
| **Puzzles** | visualization, concentration, planning and organizing, and reasoning |
| **Story/reminiscing groups** | focus, concentration, improving recall, and impulse control |
| **Card games** | memory, decision making, turn taking, concentration, focus, planning, and organizing |
| **Scavenger hunt** | focus, concentration, improving recall, and problem solving |
| **Searching and scanning games** | focus, concentration, and improving recall. |

## TYPES OF INTERVENTIONS USED TO ENCOURAGE PROCESSING SKILLS

**Processing skills** are an executive functioning skill that includes working memory, attention, and sequencing. These skills are important because they allow us to understand information that we observe and help us make judgments and show understanding of our environment. These skills can be encouraged with the following tasks:

| Activity | Skills |
|---|---|
| **jigsaw puzzles** | looking at the picture on the box and recreating it |
| **games such as Boggle, Jenga, and Taboo** | unscrambling and identifying letters, words, and shapes |
| **form constancy and figure ground handouts** | filter information, spatial perception, visual discrimination, and attention to detail |
| **visual sequential games** | visual scanning, categorizing, filter information, and identifying shapes and objects |
| **open-ended-question games or cause-and-effect question games** | reasoning, grouping skills, inference skills, decision making, executive functioning, planning, and organizing |
| **paint by numbers** | spatial perception, visual discrimination, and attention to detail. |

## ACTIVITIES USED TO FACILITATE ORAL MOTOR SKILLS FOR DRINKING, EATING, AND SWALLOWING

**Oral motor skills** involve the movement and coordination of the lips, tongue, palate, jaw, and teeth in order to complete the tasks of eating, chewing, and swallowing. As OTs, there is overlap in our scope of practice versus the scope of a speech therapist; however, we do not work on the act of swallowing with our patients. We improve feeding behaviors and eating. Some of the common strategies to facilitate oral motor skills are the following:

- blowing bubbles
- chewing gum
- use curly straws when drinking
- vibration tools
- blow with horns and whistles
- funny-face mirror games.

## INTERVENTIONS USED WITH AT-RISK YOUTH TO PROMOTE PREVOCATIONAL, VOCATIONAL, AND TRANSITIONAL SERVICES

At-risk youth are middle school-aged and high school-aged children who have not mastered basic academic, social, behavioral, work, and vocational skills in order to be successful in life and in the community and have additional risk factors associated with their home life, the correctional system, and the community. Occupational therapy in this setting continues to be an emerging area of practice. Programming for this population focuses on daily life skills, social skills, behavioral management, anger and emotional regulation, time management, job and skill development, and responsibility. Some common areas of intervention are as follows:

| Area | Examples |
|---|---|
| independent living | paying rent, doing laundry, cooking, transportation, completing homework, cooking, parenting skills, and money management |
| prevocational skills | skills needed to find a job, résumé, volunteer work, professional appearance, college and job searches, role playing, and meeting deadlines |
| social skills | appropriate social media, group interactions, employer/employee dynamics, family dynamics, and community dynamics |
| appropriate and healthy leisure and hobbies | crafting, team sports, and volunteering |
| real experiences and mentor opportunities | bringing in local entrepreneurs, field trips to businesses, police station goodwill trips, and career and job fairs. |

## COMPENSATORY STRATEGIES TEACHING PATIENTS WITH COGNITIVE AND INTELLECTUAL DEFICITS

**Compensatory strategies** are techniques and modifications that we make to a task or the environment to compensate for a disability or deficit that makes completing a task in a traditional way difficult or impossible. Some common compensatory strategies given to people with cognitive and intellectual deficits are the following:

- making lists (grocery, to-do, chores, errands)
- labeling items around the house (placing Post-its on items to know what is in a cabinet or how to use something)
- written or pictorial task plan (picture of the bed to remind patient to make the bed)
- use of mnemonics (using a fire extinguisher: PASS. **P**ull the pin. **A**im at the base of the fire. **S**queeze the trigger. **S**weep across the fire.)
- cues both verbal and visual (The patient is verbally cued to wash hands for dinner or places a sign on the fridge to wash hands before eating.)

- "chunking" (information put together into categories or small groups, for example, all morning activities: brush teeth, wash face, eat breakfast, get dressed, and use the bathroom)
- picture/name/face recall activities (putting pictures of the activity on the to-do list)
- journaling — writing down everything that needs to happen or tasks that need to be completed.

## TYPES OF ADAPTIVE INTERVENTIONS USED FOR SOMEONE WITH NEUROMOTOR DEFICITS

The term neuromotor has to do with the nerve impulses that are transmitted to muscles. **Neuromotor deficits** are seen when there is damage to the brain and spinal cord, and they will cause deficits in basic motor skills and cognition. Some of the common compensatory strategies given to people with neuromotor deficits are the following:

- **Adaptive equipment:** spike boards for meal prep, modified plates with guards and utensils that are weighted or built up, Dycem, foam to build up handles, transfer boards, walkers, wheelchairs, and shower chairs.
- **Strategy techniques:** making lists, using a calendar, using reminder functions on the phone or computer, decreasing visual and auditory stimulation, making written or picture task lists, and using energy-conservation techniques.

## WILBARGER BRUSHING PROTOCOL/DEEP PRESSURE AND PROPRIOCEPTIVE TECHNIQUE

The **Wilbarger Brushing Protocol/Deep Pressure and Proprioceptive Technique** is part of a sensory integration program that is used to treat tactile defensiveness. It involves using a soft plastic therapy brush that is moved over the child's skin using very firm pressure. Brushing starts at the arms and moves to the feet, but the brush never comes in contact with the face, chest, or stomach. The brushing protocol is generally completed every 2 hours while the child is awake and is usually followed by deep pressure at all the major joints (shoulder, hips, knees, wrist, fingers, and ankles) from the therapist or by having the child complete the joint compression by jumping and moving on his own.

## DETERMINING IF A TASK NEEDS TO BE GRADED

Grading a task is the modification of an activity to support the client's current functional performance. By altering the task's variables and continuums, you can change the difficulty of the task to meet the goals and needs of the patient. The following are examples of ways to grade an activity:

- context of the situation
- with gravity or gravity eliminated
- using verbal, tactile, or physical cues versus without cues
- timed or untimed
- one-step versus multiple-step directions
- static versus dynamic
- concrete versus abstract
- play can be solitary, parallel, cooperative, or competitive
- extrinsic versus intrinsic motivators
- eyes open versus vision occluded

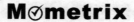

## GRADING THE THERAPEUTIC EXERCISE PROGRAM

### SOMEONE WHO NEEDS TO INCREASE ACTIVITY TOLERANCE AND ENDURANCE

You may need to grade an exercise program because of your patient's activity tolerance, precautions, or diagnosis. Grading a therapeutic exercises program can be done by altering the following:

- amount of weight
- type of weight (dumbbells, wrist weight, kettlebells, dowel stick)
- tension of exercise band
- changing from sitting to standing
- changing to active assist versus independent
- free weight versus machine (pulley system)
- timed versus untimed
- number of repetitions
- duration of the activity

### SOMEONE WITH COGNITIVE DEFICITS

A person with cognitive deficits may have difficult with their exercise program for many reasons. It could be a coordination issue, an understanding issue, or a context issue. Strengthening can still be an important component of their recovery, and it is essential for you to make the activity attainable. Grading a therapeutic exercises program for cognition can be done by altering the following:

- using handouts that have both pictures and wording
- using hand weights with Velcro or using wrist weights if they get distracted and drop the weights frequently
- training a family member or caregiver to lead the exercises for home
- doing the activity with the patient so that they have an active visual cue
- recording (video or audio) yourself explaining each activity for context and consistency
- taking pictures of the patient completing each activity and putting it into a book for their reference
- color coding each exercise station or activity
- putting signs on each activity or station
- making it a game in which a bell is rung after each task is complete

### SOMEONE WHO NEEDS TO INCREASE THEIR COORDINATION

Coordination is essential for all activity from eating to reading and functional mobility. Coordination activities are designed to facilitate coordinated, smooth, and organized movement. Grading a therapeutic program for coordination can be done by altering the following:

- transition from one side to a bilateral activity
- static ball toss to dynamic ball toss/walk-toss ball game
- changing the size of the holes in a lacing or stringing activity
- using multiple-size nuts and bolts to screw and unscrew/locks and keys of varying sizes
- contralateral/ipsilateral marching
- changing the circumference of the brush/writing utensil from small to large
- movement/functional ambulation with focal point changes
- multiple-size pill bottles and jars/varying the size of beads to place in each container

## SOMEONE WHO NEEDS TO INCREASE THEIR BALANCE

Balance is something that everyone works on from children first working on mobility to people you see at the gym working out, to seniors in fall-prevention programs. Balance activities are one of the easiest activities to grade by changing simple things. Grading a balance program can be done by altering the following:

- changing the texture of the surface (hard floor, grass, mats, gravel)
- eyes open versus occluded
- holding on for support versus hands free
- single leg versus bilateral leg
- difficulty of obstacle course (reaching high and low)
- base of support from wide to narrow
- contralateral/ipsilateral ambulation and static balance
- static and dynamic balance with focal point changes
- mobility with reading or/and with focal point changes
- standing on a trampoline for functional activity

## SOMEONE WHO NEEDS TO INCREASE THEIR FLEXIBILITY

ADLs and functional mobility can be difficult because of deficits in flexibility. Limited flexibility can be caused by scar tissue, edema, age, activity levels, and internal body structures. Grading a flexibility program can be done by altering the following:

- Tai Chi/yoga can be modified to sitting or standing
- water stretching class/activity versus on land
- stretching standing versus sitting
- using physical agent modalities (PAMs) to warm the muscles before exercise
- passive range of motion (PROM) versus active range of motion (AROM)
- isometric activity
- hold/relax stretch techniques.

## FACILITATING PARTICIPATION IN A GROUP WHEN A PATIENT DOES NOT WANT TO ENGAGE

Group tasks and activities are important because they promote cooperation, interaction, socialization, working as a team, and comradery, which are skills needed to be a successful and active member of the community, at work, and in life. It can also cause group members to be more productive, creative, and motivated in completing tasks. There are many strategies to encourage participation when a patient does not want to engage:

- Don't force participation or compromise. The client may not want to stay for the group, so allow observation or partial participation for a set amount of time.
- Build rapport and use positive feedback. If clients trust you, they will often participate, and pointing out their strengths is a great motivator.
- Find their purpose. During your evaluation you should have determined the client's motivation when setting goals. An activity group that is addressing UE exercises and gross motor tasks may seem boring, but when given perspective to the task and how it relates to the patient's overall goal, participation may make more sense and be more likely.

## TYPE OF INTERVENTIONS USED TO INCREASE UE STRENGTH IN YOUR PATIENT

To increase UE strength in your patient, you can use traditional weighted exercises or use more therapeutic activity based on the needs of your patient. The following are interventions used to increase arm strength:

- dumbbells, kettlebells, TheraBand, arm weights
- arm bike/upper body ergometer
- dowel stick exercises
- chair/wall or kneeing pushups
- medicine ball or weighted ball toss
- seated leaning into side lying with arm support
- planks
- folding laundry, organizing canned goods in a pantry, gardening, and making the bed

## TYPE OF INTERVENTIONS USED TO INCREASE THE ROM IN YOUR PATIENT

ROM exercises help maintain mobility and flexibility and help improve joint function. These activities are important for everyone, not just people recovering from injury because they can improve circulation, reduce stiffness and pain, and decrease the likelihood of injury. The only contraindications to ROM stretches are hypermobility of the joint, inflammation or infection, and an unstable joint. The following are interventions used to increase ROM:

- Passive range of motion (PROM): The therapist, family, or equipment moves the joint through its range with no assist form the patient.
- Active assist range of motion (AAROM): The patient only exerts minimal effort to help the therapist, family, or equipment move the joint through its range.
- Active range of motion (AROM): The patient is able to move the joint through its full range independently.
- Proprioceptive neuromuscular facilitation stretching techniques are series of movements that allow the muscles to stretch farther than what's achievable with a normal stretch or ROM activity. The muscle is stretched, and this is followed by an isometric contraction. This can reduce muscle tone and allow for a better stretch and a fuller ROM in the joint.
- Specifically, for shoulder ROM, use pulleys, wall walking/wall ladders, wall/table "washing," arm bike, and arm clocks.

## TYPE OF INTERVENTIONS USED TO INCREASE ACTIVITY TOLERANCE IN YOUR PATIENT

**Activity** tolerance is the amount of physical activity that a person can tolerate and complete before adverse vitals and fatigue are felt. Activity tolerance is measured respiration rate, blood pressure, heart rate, and oxygen levels as well as observing physical signs such as pallor and perspiration. Vital signs are measured before the activity starts, during the activity, immediately at the conclusion of the activity, and again 5 minutes after the activity is concluded to determine if the vitals have returned to baseline. Activity tolerance is a significant part of treatment for patients with cardiac and respiratory issues, and the ability to grade tasks becomes a key component. The following are interventions used to increase activity tolerance:

- upper body ergometer/arm bike
- simple ADLs: gathering supplies and then standing for dressing/grooming, simple meal prep, folding and putting away laundry, and sweeping or washing windows
- standing while completing puzzles, board games, drawing, and balloon volley
- scavenger hunts with bending and reaching activities.

## TYPE OF INTERVENTIONS USED TO DESENSITIZE NERVE PAIN IN YOUR PATIENT

Patients who have had surgery or an injury that affects the nerves can often have hypersensitivity to the most basic stimuli in that area, and a desensitization program needs to be created. This process needs to start slow and work into something your patient can tolerate. It may begin with the stimuli being introduced less than 30 seconds at a time. Using a timer is key with these interventions to show increasing tolerance. These activities should be completed up to five times a day.

- Contrast bath. Use a container of cold water (45°F to 70°F) and a container of warm water (104°F to 110°F). Place the area of injury in the cold container for 30 seconds then into the warm container for 2 minutes at a time. Do this five times and finish in the warm water.
- Fabric touch. Take various types of fabric with different textures (cotton, silk, felt) and lightly rub the affected area.
- Rice and sand bins. Have the affected area in the textures moving or touching items hidden in the bins.
- Vibration. Use vibrating devices along the affected areas.
- Rolling. Use a foam roller or small smooth and textured balls to roll over the area. Small painting rollers work well.

## TYPE OF INTERVENTIONS USED TO INCREASE POSTURAL CONTROL IN YOUR PATIENT

**Postural control** is the ability of the body to position itself in relation to the task or activity that is being completed. Having a strong core improves postural control, which directly affects the use of our arms to reach, grasp, and complete tasks. The following are interventions used to increase postural control:

- sitting on a therapy ball and making small side-to-side and circular movements with the hips (can be graded by moving the feet from a wide to a narrow stance)
- playing games, reading, and activities in prone
- yoga and Tai Chi movements and classes
- sit-to-stand activities
- for children, the use of animal walks and pumping on a swing
- household chores such as vacuuming and carrying laundry baskets
- throwing balls of multiple sizes and weights and playing balloon volley using pool noodles as a bat.

## TYPE OF INTERVENTIONS USED TO INCREASE BALANCE IN YOUR PATIENT

**Balance** is the ability to stay upright while maintaining control and coordination of the body, and it can be static or dynamic. Static balance is the ability to maintain postural stability in one place. Dynamic balance is the ability to maintain postural stability with movement. Balance is at the core of all functional movement and activity. As we age, balance becomes more problematic with the Centers for Disease Control and Prevention reporting that one in five falls will cause a serious injury. Our balance can be affected by our environment (loose rugs, slips on ice, and trips on cords) our health (medications, high blood pressure, vertigo) and can be strictly an accident (dog tripped you on a walk). The following are interventions that are used to increase balance:

- heel-toe walking
- obstacle courses involving change of direction, stepping over items, and reaching
- Tai Chi and yoga
- standing LE strengthening (heel and toe lifts, knee bends, and mini lunges)

- standing on one foot, balance boards
- completing functional tasks, changing stance from wide to narrow.
- arm exercises while seated on a wobble cushion or therapy ball.

## DEVELOPING PROGRAMS

### SOMEONE WHO NEEDS NEUROMUSCULAR REEDUCATION

**Neuromuscular reeducation** is used to help a patient regain normal movement after a stroke, trauma, or brain injury, and it is a type of treatment modality in conjunction with the regular therapy session. During the evaluation process, you take a detailed history with close attention to the symptoms that your patient is having. You will assess strength, muscle tone, balance, joint mobility, posture, fine motor ability, and sensation in addition to ADLs, use of equipment, and functional mobility as you would in any evaluation. The program will be based on the evaluation findings and will focus on repetitive movement, posturing, and using different types of stimulation to elicit and reinforce signals from the nerves to the muscles in functional activity. The goal of neuromuscular reeducation is retraining the nerve signals to create the appropriate movement consistently until the movement becomes automatic.

### SOMEONE WHO NEEDS PAIN MANAGEMENT

**Pain management** is often a part of therapy sessions, even if that is not the primary reason that a patient is coming to you. Pain can be from an old issue or injury, or it could be directly related to the reason that the patient is seeing you. It is required by Medicare and most insurance companies that a pain assessment is completed for every interaction with your patient. Chronic pain can lead to loss of mobility, decreased ADLs, decreased independence, and difficulty with work, home, and social interactions and can lead to medication dependency. In addition to the activities and interventions that you put in place for the primary problem, the following are intervention approaches for pain management:

- relaxation and mediation techniques including deep breathing
- body mechanics and ergonomics for daily activities that may be triggering pain
- regulating and pacing activities to avoid pain flare-ups
- a HEP that includes stretching activities
- therapeutic taping/splinting for pain
- PAMs
- neuromuscular reeducation
- coping strategies

### SOMEONE WHO NEEDS EDEMA REDUCTION

**Edema** can be caused by many reasons including medications, postsurgical swelling, disease process, injury, lack of mobility, and obesity. It can lead to decreased function in all areas of life and can even cause pain. Once the cause of the edema is determined and contraindications are ruled out, the therapeutic process can begin. During the initial evaluation, measurements, pictures, sensation, and pitting are noted specifically in the edematous area in addition to the typical evaluation format so that progress can be noted throughout each session. Specific interventions to address edema are as follows:

- manual joint mobilization and retrograde massage
- exercises and activities designed to decrease edema
- fitting and education of don/doff and care of compression garments/bandages
- skin care

- continuous passive motion (CPM) machine
- diet (including reading labels to determine salt intake)
- e-stim

## SOMEONE WHO NEEDS SCAR MANAGEMENT AND MOBILIZATION

Scars can be a result of recent surgery, burns, traumatic injury, or as part of the disease process. In addition to the typical evaluation, pictures and measurements of the scar must be taken and a home exercises program is recommended for carryover techniques. Patients are advised to complete self-scar massage two or three times a day for up to 10 minutes at a time and to moisturize the scar daily to keep it pliable. Specific interventions to address scar management are as follows:

- nutrition/diet education to promote healing
- scar massage (hands-on/vibration)
- compression therapy (bandages, garments, mechanical)
- topical treatments (silicone gel)
- PAMs (paraffin and ultrasound)
- exercises and activities to promote mobilization of the scar
- splinting to avoid contractures
- skin care
- desensitization activity
- sensory and neuromuscular reeducation

## SOMEONE WHO NEEDS TO IMPROVE OVERALL BODY MECHANICS AND POSTURAL STABILITY

**Body mechanics** is the ability of muscles to maintain body posture stability in standing or performing tasks. Proper body mechanics allows us to move in a task or activity in a way that will avoid injury. The most common injury we see due to poor body mechanics is from not lifting items safely using the legs versus using the muscles of the back. During the evaluation process, we want to find specific details about the patient's daily life and work activities so that we can recreate as many true-to-life scenarios in the clinic for training. Proper lifting body mechanics require you to bend at the hips and not the waist, have your feet stabilized and aligned with your hips underneath you, and keep your neck and trunk aligned while lifting the item close to your body. We also want to train our patients to pull rather than push an object to avoid strain on the back. In addition to teaching the proper mechanics, we will provide exercises for strengthening and flexibility of the hips, back, and arms.

## SOMEONE WHO NEEDS TO IMPROVE STRESS MANAGEMENT WITH BREATHING PATTERNS AND TECHNIQUES

Occupational therapy is holistic in nature, and we are trained to treat the whole person, not just the disease or disability. This helps us in our treatment planning because many of our patients come to us feeling anxious, scared, sad, angry, and overwhelmed because of the disease process or injury that they are seeing us for. Managing stress and anxiety often becomes part of our treatment plan despite the treating diagnosis. In addition to exploring hobbies and leisure pursuits to address these concerns, it is well within our scope of practice to educate our patients in deep-breathing techniques, progressive muscle relaxation, and guided imagery and add to these to the goals in the plan of care.

- Deep-breathing techniques: Use diaphragmatic breathing and pursed-lip breathing.
- Progressive muscle relaxation: The patient starts distally at the feet and works up and then back to the feet again by tightening each muscle group for 5 seconds and then releasing the contraction. At the conclusion of the activity, the whole body relaxes completely.

- Guided imagery: Using words and music, lead your patient on a relaxing mental journey using specific descriptive words to stimulate the senses. (As you walk along the beach, feel the warm, damp sand and the gentle waves touch your ankles as the water comes ashore. Can you smell the water and the faint scent of sunscreen in the air?)

## ISOTONIC, ISOKINETIC, AND ISOMETRIC EXERCISES

Muscle contraction can be divided into three categories: isotonic, isokinetic, and isometric. **Isotonic contractions** cause the muscle to change in length as it contracts. There are two types of isotonic contractions: concentric and eccentric. **Concentric contractions** cause the muscle to shorten as it contracts. **Eccentric contractions** are the opposite of concentric and are when the muscle lengthens during contraction. Isokinetic contractions also cause the muscle to change in length during the contraction but also produces movements of a constant speed. **Isometric contractions** are when there is no change in the length of the muscle that is contracting. The following are examples of isotonic, isokinetic, and isometric exercises:

| Category | Exercise |
| --- | --- |
| Isotonic | Muscles maintain the same tension throughout the exercise: bicep curls, squats, lunges, push-ups, bench presses, sit-ups, pulleys, therapy bands. |
| Isokinetic | The resistance and speed of the exercise are controlled with machines, and it provides variable resistance despite the level of exertion. Bike, dynamometers, and exercise machines. |
| Isometric | Does not move muscles through a range of movement and keeps them stable. Plank, yoga, wall sit, bridging, and wall exercises. |

## COMMON ARM INJURIES

**Radial tunnel syndrome** and **cubital tunnel syndrome** are caused by nerve compression in the wrist, arm, and elbow. Both cause numbness and tingling in the hands and fingers. **Lateral epicondylitis**, also known as tennis elbow, is inflammation of the tendons that attach the forearm muscles to the outside of the elbow. **Medial epicondylitis**, also known as golfer's elbow, is inflammation of the tendons that attach the forearm muscles to the inside of the elbow. Both are caused by repetitive, aggressive, forceful gripping and lifting movements and are most often seen in people that have skilled-trade jobs and do factory work.

### RADIAL TUNNEL SYNDROME

**Symptoms**: Aching at the forearm below the elbow. Can cause a sharp stabbing pain with flexion of the wrist and fingers. Fatigue and muscle weakness in the arm.

**Cause**: The radial nerve is compressed as it travels through the elbow. Caused by repetitive movement twisting the arm or wrist, gripping, and hand manipulation.

**Treatment**: Splinting, wrist strap, nerve gliding, and strengthening exercises.

### CUBITAL TUNNEL SYNDROME

**Symptoms**: Numbness and tingling in the ring finger and the little finger. Causes fine motor and dexterity deficits.

**Cause**: The ulnar nerve is compressed in the elbow. Caused by pressure or leaning on the elbow when it is bent, sustained time with a bent elbow, talking on the phone, curling your hand under your pillow when you sleep.

**Treatment**: Splinting to keep the elbow straight, nerve gliding, and strengthening exercises.

## LATERAL EPICONDYLITIS/TENNIS ELBOW

**Symptoms**: Weak grip strength, pain and burning in the elbow, difficulty gripping and twisting, and pain from the lateral elbow down the arm to the hand.

**Cause**: Inflammation of a tendon from overuse.

**Treatment**: Therapy tape, elbow brace, splinting, exercise, PAMs, strengthening and stretching exercises, rest, and nerve and tendon gliding exercises.

## MEDIAL EPICONDYLITIS/GOLFER'S ELBOW

**Symptoms**: Weakness in the hands and wrists, numbness and tingles in the hand and fingers, and pain in the medial elbow down the arm to the hand.

**Cause**: Inflammation of a tendon from overuse.

**Treatment**: Therapy tape, elbow brace, splinting, exercise, PAMs, strengthening and stretching exercises, rest, and nerve and tendon gliding exercises.

## DUPUYTREN'S CONTRACTURE, DE QUERVAIN'S TENOSYNOVITIS, AND TRIGGER FINGER

Dupuytren's contracture, De Quervain's tenosynovitis, and trigger finger all involve the tendons of the hand. Treatment is similar in all three conditions: rest, tendon gliding exercises, PAMs, and splinting; the physician may include a steroid shot into the tendon sheath as a last possibility before surgery is indicated.

- **Dupuytren's contracture** is caused by an abnormal thickening of the tissues in the palm between the skin and the tendons, giving the appearance of cords. The thickening will eventually cause the fingers to be pulled into the palm into a bent position.
- **De Quervain's** tenosynovitis is caused when the tendons around the base of the thumb become swollen, causing the sheaths that cover the tendons to become inflamed. This compresses the nerves, causing pain, tingling, and numbness.
- **Trigger finger** is an inflammation in the tendons of the finger, often brought on by overuse or repetitive movement and complications with gout, diabetes, and arthritis. If it is not treated, the affected finger can become permanently locked in the bent position. Symptoms include a nodule or lump at the base of the finger, popping/clicking with movement, and the affected digit getting stuck in a bent position, requiring the patient to physically straighten the finger with the other hand.

## GALVESTON BRACING AND A GIVMOHR SLING

A **Galveston brace** is used when there are fractures of the second through fifth metacarpal bones. This is called a boxer's fracture and is most often seen as a result of a fight. This brace has a three-point fixation and allows for unrestricted movement of the IP, metacarpophalangeal (MP), and wrist joint. A **GivMohr sling** is used for functional positioning of the UE in a flaccid arm as well as joint compression during standing and ambulation. It is most commonly used in post stroke patients to help avoid subluxation of the shoulder joint.

## MUSCLES MAKING UP THE ROTATOR CUFF

The four muscles that make up the rotator cuff (RTC) are the **supraspinatus muscle**, **infraspinatus muscle**, **teres minor muscle**, and **subscapularis muscle**. The mnemonic to remember these is SITS. The RTC lifts and rotates the arm and stabilizes the head of the humerus in the socket of the joint. Tears in these muscles often come from a fall in older adults, but they can also be caused by lifting heavy items or repetitive overhead motions. Tears can be partial or complete. In a partial tear, the tendon of the RTC is damaged, but it is not completely severed or torn. In a complete tear, the muscle is torn into two separate pieces or completely torn off of the humerus. RTC tears can often be treated nonsurgically with anti-inflammatory medication; steroid injections; and therapy for ADL modifications, ROM, and strengthening. If surgery is required, the surgeon will provide protocols with specific ROM guidelines post-surgery and therapy will consist of ADL modifications, basic isometric exercises, pendulum exercises, PAMs, and PROM/active assisted range of motion (AAROM) with scapula elevations and retractions and no weights for the first 6 weeks. When the patient is cleared by the surgeon, light resistance with increasing repetitions, AROM, and strengthening will begin.

## AMPUTATION

A patient with a new amputation has had their life significantly changed. In addition to working on mobility and ADLs, there are also the psychosocial and emotional damage to deal with, and each person reacts very differently. Working through a sense of loss, self-worth, and self-esteem often become major pieces of the treatment plan. Amputations can be caused from trauma (military deployment injuries, motor vehicle accidents), tumors, infections, and systemic issues (diabetic complications, circulation issues, peripheral vascular disease [PVD], arteriosclerosis, and venous insufficiency). LE amputations are more common than UE amputations. Amputations are designated by joint level in most cases. In the UE: above elbow, below elbow (short, medium or long), and phalangeal amputation. In the LE: hemipelvectomy (complete hip), above knee (short, middle, or supracondylar), below knee (short, medium, or long), Syme amputation (just above the ankle), transmetatarsal, and toe amputations.

### AMPUTATION SURGICAL PROCESS

Amputation surgery can be closed or open. Closed amputation is when the tissue is in good shape and can be used to completely close the wound using skin flaps. In an open amputation, there is usually an infection or compromised skin, and the wound is left open to allow the infection to clear. Often, a wound VAC is placed to help the healing process. A second surgery will be needed after the infection is cleared in order to close the wound. The stitches/staples are generally removed within 3 to 4 weeks of the procedure. Patients are fit for limb shrinkers at that time and need to wear them at all times until the initial prosthesis is fit.

## PROSTHESIS

Once the residual limb has healed after amputation, the process of getting a prosthetic begins. When the stitches are removed and the wound is healed, the patient is fit for a limb shrinker by an orthotist. The limb shrinker reduces edema, helps reshape the stump, reduces phantom limb issues, acts as a desensitizer, and helps with pain management. Part of the treatment plan at this point is making sure there is proper skin care to the stump, teaching how to check for breakdown and wounds, and that the patient can clean the limb shrinker as well as get it on and off easily. An impression of the limb will be taken, and a check socket is made. A check socket helps create a proper fitting prosthesis because the socket is the part of the prosthesis where the residual limb sits. A temporary prosthesis is made that allows the patient to begin ambulating. It can be altered easily as the edema changes in the stump and allows for specifics about socket design and aesthetics to be figured out before a final prosthetic is created. The initial prosthesis is worn for up to 6 months. When the final prosthetic is in place, the orthotist ensures proper fitting and does initial gait training. At that point, PT and OT begin to work on more detailed activity for ADLs and functional mobility.

## CONTUSIONS, CRUSH INJURIES, AND DISLOCATIONS

Contusions, crush injuries, and dislocations are common occurrences in a traumatic event, natural disaster, or accident.

| Condition | Definition |
| --- | --- |
| Contusion | A type of hematoma also known as a bruise, which is caused when blood vessels are damaged or broken. A patient can have a skin or a bone contusion. |
| Crush injury | Caused when a part of the body is pressed and squeezed between two objects. People with traumatic soft-tissue injury are at risk of developing rhabdomyolysis, which is death of muscle that releases protein into the bloodstream triggering kidney failure. |
| Dislocation | A dislocation is an injury in which a bone or joint is dislodged from alignment. Causes pain, tingling, and loss of movement as the muscles are pulled out of place when the bone dislodges. |

## SPRAIN VS. STRAIN

A sprain and a strain are each soft-tissue injuries. These injuries are caused by trauma or overuse in the muscles, tendons, and ligaments. A sprain is the overstretching of ligaments, and a strain is the overstretching of muscles and tendons. Both conditions can be placed in one of three categories based on the severity of the injury.

| Category | Definition |
| --- | --- |
| Grade 1 (mild) | Minimal edema, painful to touch, slight microscopic tearing of fibers, minimal overstretching. Recovery is 1–2 weeks. |
| Grade 2 (moderate) | Moderate edema and pain, unable to support weight through the affected area, moderate but not complete tearing of fibers. Recovery is 3–4 weeks. |
| Grade 3 (severe) | Significant pain and swelling, unable to bear weight, joint is unstable, complete tear and rupture of fibers. Recovery can be 4–8 weeks based on the severity of the injury and other factors such as age, previous injuries, and activity levels. |

## TYPES OF SHOULDER FRACTURES

A shoulder fracture can be caused by a fall, trauma, or even a sports injury. These fractures will involve a break to the clavicle, the proximal end of the humerus, or the scapula. If the fractures are minor, they can be treated without surgery, which is considered a closed reduction. The patient will wear a shoulder immobilizer sling for several weeks to allow the weight of the arm to keep traction aligning the bone fragments while they heal. If the break is more serious, surgery may be indicated called an open reduction internal fixation, in which the bone is repaired with a metal plate and screws. If the damage is significant and the bone is unable to be repaired, a patient will need a hemiarthroplasty, which is a replacement of the proximal humerus with an artificial joint. The first 2–4 weeks of therapy will only consist of pendulum exercises; AROM/PROM of the elbow, wrist, hand, and finger; PROM of the shoulder in the plane of the scapula; scapular isometric exercises (protraction, retraction, elevation, and depression); and modalities for edema, muscle relaxation, and pain management. The patient is not allowed any internal or external rotation of the shoulder. At 6 weeks post-surgery/injury, therapy can begin with PROM/AROM/AAROM of the shoulder, elbow, wrist, and hand and isometric rotator cuff strengthening exercises adding in isotonic strengthening as tolerated. Aggressive UE strengthening exercises will begin at the 10-week mark.

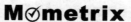

## JOINT MOBILIZATION VS. JOINT MANIPULATION

**Joint mobilization** is very specific movement performed by a therapist of the articular surfaces of the joint to decrease pain and increase joint mobility. It is considered to be a form of PROM. It is performed slowly with no stretching movement and is designed to restore the normal joint play that has been compromised by injury. **Joint manipulation** is also a type of PROM provided by a therapist that involves the manipulation of a joint, using thrusting maneuvers that produces a popping sound. It is provided for pain relief, increase of range of motion, and to "unstick" or "release" a stiff joint.

## SPLINTING

**Splinting** is an orthopedic procedure in which a device is fabricated to protect, control pain, immobilize, and support a broken bone or injured tendon, muscle, or ligament. They can be fabricated by a therapist, or they can be prefabricated and off the shelf and ordered based on the injury, body part, or category of the splint (for example, a resting hand splint). They can be modified and adjusted based on the amount of edema that is present, which is why they are often used first after surgery prior to a traditional plaster cast. Splints may be static, dynamic, or static progressive.

- **Considerations:** Diagnosis, age, splint design, ability to don/doff with ease, comfort, environment, purpose, occupational performance needs, wearing schedule, friability of skin
- **Contraindications/Complication:** Contraindicated: excessive swelling, neurovascular compromise.
- **Complications**: compartment syndrome, pressure ulcer.
- **Thermoplastic Splinting Materials:** Most common for custom splint, low temperature/soften in water at 135°F–180°F. Can drape on the patient to mold when warm. Standard is 1/8-inch-thick, with multiple colors and patterns.
- **Positive/Negative for Prefabricated Splints:**
  o   Pros: Buy at most drug stores, minimal self-adjustments, and easy to take on and off.
  o   Cons: Difficult to keep clean, comes in basic sizes (small, medium, and large).
- **Positive/Negative for Custom Splints:**
  o   Pros: They are made out of thermoplastic material and cut and fit specifically to the patient. Can be adjusted and altered as needed with a heat gun. Easy to clean.
  o   Cons: Labor intensive to make. Do not hold up if left in a hot car.

Splinting is used to immobilize and support and injured area. There are three types of splinting: static, dynamic, and static progressive. **Static splinting** is used for positioning, support, and immobilizing the area. This splint does not move. **Dynamic splinting** is often spring loaded and is used to increase ROM. **Static progressive splinting** is when the splint is adjustable using nonelastic pieces to apply torque to a joint in order to position it as close to the end range as possible, increasing the PROM. An **outrigger** is a piece attached to a splint that allows traction for the fingers as well as an anchor for mobilizing force and a 90-degree angle of pull. Outriggers can be high or low profile. A **high-profile outrigger** is a deviation from the 90-degree pull, whereas a **low-profile outrigger** is a greater deviation from the 90-degree pull.

### SPLINTING MATERIAL OPTIONS

Splinting material comes in many categories. Most splinting material traditionally comes in sheets that are 18″ × 24″ and are 1/16″, 3/32″, 1/8″, and 3/16″ thick. The conformability and resistance to stretch can range from minimum to moderate to maximum resistant. Splint materials can vary by memory, amount of drape, bonding, rigidity, and perforated or solid; they come in almost any color or pattern. A single type of material does not work for all splints. Every splinting material is different, but the optimal heating temperature is from 140°–170°F with up to a 2-minute heating time and a working time of 1–7 minutes.

## ESSENTIAL PIECES OF EQUIPMENT NEEDED FOR SPLINTING

In order to fabricate a splint, there are essential pieces of equipment you need access to. They are as follows:

- **Heating source**
  - Splint pan.
  - Heat gun.
  - You can use a hydrocollator if you have no other option, but this is not ideal because you can't control the water temperature and may overstretch the material.
- **Splint tools**
  - Cutting device (scissors, utility knife).
  - Pliers and wire cutters (for manipulating outriggers).
  - Hole punches (for outriggers, hinges, and strapping)
  - Hand drill (to make holes too deep for the hand punch or to add perforations to the material).
  - Plastic spatula/tongs (to manipulate the material in the water).
  - A towel or sheet to rest the material on when it is removed out of the water and dry off the excess water.
  - Grease pen to mark areas of concern or indentations that need to be made and molded and paper towels to fabricate a pattern.
  - Always protect the patient's hand with a stockinette.

## GOALS

The **goals of splinting** are as follows:

- rest and support of the injured area
- stabilize and protect the injured area
- increase or protect ROM
- positioning
- facilitate or deter movement
- increase functional activity and movement

## BIOMECHANICS

The **biomechanics of splinting** are as follows:

- increase the area of force (wider splints, uniform pressure, rolled edges)
- increase the mechanical advantage (splints are first-class levers, larger forearm trough, proximal and distal strap placement)
- three-point fixation (decrease pressure with wide diagonal straps, proximal and distal counterforces, and two parallel forces)
- abrupt pressure transitions (where the splint ends or transitions, edges need to be flared, straps rounded, and straps and padding need to be diagonal and soft)
- stress concentration (even pressure and contouring of the splint)
- friction (poor fastening devices, bad joint alignment, bad fitting)

## FITTING A SPLINT PROPERLY

Splinting is a good way to stabilize and support an injury, and it is often a better option than casting because a splint is noncircumferential and allows swelling without the pressure-related complications and skin breakdown often caused by casting. The considerations when splinting are as follows:

- Biomechanics (splinting is a lever).
- Be aware of and accommodate bony prominences.
- Understand and maintain the arches of the hand.
- Do not block uninvolved joints (inhibit movement in a functioning joint).
- Rounded corners and smooth edges when fabricating will prevent skin issues.
- Be mindful of wrist position and the ability of the fingers to move.

## FABRICATION PROCESS IN SPLINTING

When you are tasked with making a custom splint for a patient, use the word **PROCESS** to remember the areas to address in order to complete the splint.

- **P**: Pattern creation: Mark the border and make sure to leave a half inch around the edges for proper edging.
- **R**: Refine the pattern: Make sure that the joint motion you want is allowed and that the lateral borders are wide enough to prevent unwanted compression from the strapping.
- **O**: Options for material: What works best for your patient — perforated plastic, thin material, the ability to be remolded often?
- **C**: Cut and heat: Try to position the patient's hand on the material and use Coban or another type of wrap on the patient's hand to protect the skin during the molding process.
- **E**: Evaluate the fit when molding the splint: Looking at stability and changing the shape, determining where things need to flare or require padding. This is a fluid, ever-changing process during molding.
- **S**: Strapping and components: Strap to secure the splint; apply thin straps between the fingers to avoid bulk padding.
- **S**: Splint finishing touches: Check to see if the splint does what it was intended to do, smooth out marks and fingerprints you may have left, smooth the edges, and round the tabs of the strapping.

## HAND AND FINGER SPLINTS

Hand and finger splinting can be an exciting and creative area for a therapist to find their niche in a facility or community by designing custom splints and splint patterns in addition to tailoring prefabricated splints. These are the four main categories for hand and finger splinting. If an area is too awkward or it is cumbersome for a splint, tape is used as an alternative.

| Category | Use |
|---|---|
| Ulnar gutter | Used for positioning in RA or OA and used for soft-tissue injuries and fractures to the ring and small fingers. Supports the mid forearm on the ulnar side to the distal interphalangeal joint (DIP) of the ring and small fingers. |
| Radial gutter | Used for positioning in RA or OA and used for soft-tissue injuries and fractures to the index and middle fingers. Supports the mid forearm on the radial side to the DIP of the index and middle fingers. |
| Thumb spica | Used for positioning for De Quervain's tenosynovitis, fractures in the first metacarpal, scaphoid, and lunate bones and injury to the ulnar collateral ligament. Supports the thumb in neutral and can extend from the wrist crease to mid forearm. |
| Finger splints | Used to stabilize the proximal interphalangeal (PIP), DIP, and interphalangeal (IP) joints. Also used for pain management from arthritis and to treat boutonniere finger, mallet finger, and trigger finger. Can vary in size and construction. |
| Buddy taping | Used when a fracture or sprain is difficult to cast or splint on its own. The injured finger is taped to the adjacent finger for protection and stability and to allow movement. |

## FOREARM SPLINTS

Wrist and forearm splints are used to relieve carpal tunnel and RA symptoms; stabilize fractures in the hand and wrist including fractures in the ring, index, and middle fingers; and support soft-tissue injuries. Elbow and forearm splints are used to stabilize elbow fractures and proximal radius and ulnar fractures that require the wrist and elbow to be stabilized. The following are the most common type of forearm splints:

| Category | Use |
|---|---|
| Volar short arm splint | Extends from the middle of the forearm to the distal palmar crease on the palm side of the forearm, wrist, and hand with the wrist slightly extended. |
| Dorsal short arm splint | Extends from the middle of the forearm to the distal palmar crease to the top of the forearm, wrist, and hand with the wrist slightly extended. |
| Single sugar-tong splint | Extends from the proximal palmar crease to the forearm. It covers under the elbow and the forearm, and it ends at the base of the fingers. It is most commonly used for a fracture to the radius or ulna. |
| Long arm posterior splint | Extends down the underside of the arm while the arm is bent at 90°. The trough extends from the axilla to the proximal palmar crease. It is used to stabilize fractures in the humerus near the elbow, radius, or ulna near the elbow, a fracture to the olecranon process, and any type of ligament damage in the elbow. |
| Double sugar-tong splint | The elbow is bent at a 90° angle with a splint that extends from the elbow down the forearm on the top and bottom until it reaches the base of the fingers. It is used for stabilizing Colles' fractures, fractures in the humerus near the elbow, radius, or ulna near the elbow, and fractures to the olecranon process. |

## ARCHES AND CREASES OF THE HAND AND THE COMMON PRESSURE POINTS SEEN IN SPLINTING

The three arches of the hand are the longitudinal arch, distal transverse arch, and proximal transverse arch. The longitudinal arch gives the hand the ability to flex and extend the fingers. The distal transverse arch allows the palm to flatten as the hand opens. The proximal transverse arch is rigid and is located at the carpals making up the distal end of the carpal tunnel. The creases of the hand are the distal palmar crease, proximal palmar crease, and the thenar crease. The hand creases are the axes of motion for the joint. It is important to pay attention to the creases and arches because if you splint the hand into a flat position and compromise these structures, the functional grasp and mobility are significantly limited. The common areas to watch for pressure points and skin breakdown in the wrist and hand are at the ulnar styloid, distal radial styloid, and the carpometacarpal joint in the thumb. This is because these are bony prominences and the bones are close to the skin surface, putting pressure on the skin from within and rubbing against the splint on the outside, causing the skin to break down.

## FRAMES OF REFERENCE FOR SPLINTING

The frames of reference used in splinting are compensatory, biomechanical, rehabilitation, and sensory motor. Compensatory is about increasing **functional performance** and creating independence by using compensatory techniques. Biomechanical is based on joint ROM, muscle strength, and endurance and uses the properties and principles of kinesiology and force acting on the body. Rehabilitation is based on regaining function and compensating for deficits to achieve maximum functional potential. Sensory motor is used to inhibit and facilitate normal motor responses.

## EDUCATING PATIENTS ON SPLINT CARE

When the splint is created, the patient should not leave the facility without having the splint checked multiple times for rubbing and pressure points so that it can be modified before returning home. The patient should complete skin checks every 30 minutes for comfort and pressure points when at home. Prior to leaving the session, the patient needs to be comfortable donning/doffing the splint. He should be aware of landmarks and markings on the straps for proper placement. He should be educated on how often he needs to clean the splint and techniques for cleaning including having an extra stockinette as a barrier between his skin and the splint. Finally, a wearing schedule should be in place with specific times for when the splint needs to be worn and taken off. Initially, the schedule may need to be modified to build up wearing tolerance and compliance.

## UNIVERSAL CUFFS AND TENODESIS SPLINTS

A **universal cuff** is a device that slides over the hand so that a patient with limited grip or dexterity can hold onto a writing or eating utensil. **Tenodesis** is the reciprocal motion of the wrist and fingers that happens during active or passive wrist flexion and extension. Wrist extension will cause finger flexion, and wrist flexion will cause finger extension. A tenodesis splint is used by patients with spinal cord injuries at the C6–C7 level for functional grasp.

## CLASSIFICATIONS OF NERVE INJURIES

There are three types of peripheral nerve injuries. They can be caused by stretching, lacerations, and compression. **Stretch-related injuries** are when the force on the nerve is too strong, causing it to pull or tear. **Laceration injuries** are when the nerve is severed, and these can happen by accident or from a medical procedure. A **compression injury** is when the nerve is compressed or entrapped by another structure. Peripheral nerve injuries can further be classified using the Seddon classification system. This system classifies nerve injuries into three major groups: **neurapraxia** (myelin damage caused by compression and temporary loss of motor and sensory function; lasts up to 2 months before regenerating on its own), **axonotmesis** (the axon and myelin sheath are damaged or severed but the endoneurium is intact and will likely allow regeneration), and **neurotmesis** (complete and total damage of the nerve, sheath, and trunk; will need surgical intervention).

## MEDIAN NERVE

Compression of the median nerve can cause numbness, tingling, and pain in the hands. Compression of the nerve within the carpal tunnel is the cause of carpal tunnel syndrome.

| | |
|---|---|
| **Nerve root origin** | Comes from the medial and lateral portions of the brachial plexus and originates from C6–T1. |
| **Major branches** | The anterior interosseous nerve supplies the deep muscles in the anterior forearm.<br>The palmar cutaneous nerve innervates the skin of the lateral palm. |
| **Motor function** | Innervates the flexor and pronator muscles in the anterior compartment, the thenar muscles, and the lateral two lumbricals of the hand. |
| **Sensory function** | Develops into the digital and palmar cutaneous branches that innervate the lateral palm and small, ring, and middle fingers with half of the index finger on the anterior surface of the hand. |
| **Clinical sign: high lesion** | Sensory loss, ulnar flexion of the wrist, loss of pronation, and palmar abduction/opposition. |
| **Clinical sign: low lesion** | Sensory loss, loss of opposition, thenar eminence, and palmar abduction. |
| **Treatments** | Splinting, PROM, adaptive equipment to assist with functional grip, and modification and adaptive techniques for loss of sensation. |

## ULNAR NERVE

The ulnar nerve communicates sensation and motor function through the elbow and hand. Numbness and tingling in the ring and little fingers are often the result of ulnar nerve issues.

| | |
|---|---|
| **Nerve root origin** | A peripheral nerve that originates in the brachial plexus and is a continuation of the medial cord coming from C8–T1. |
| **Major branches** | Divides two heads of the flexor carpi ulnaris and follows ulna until it branches into three parts: Muscular branch innervates muscles in anterior compartment, palmar cutaneous branch innervates skin of medial palm, and dorsal cutaneous branch innervates skin of medial index finger and palm area. |
| **Motor function** | Innervates flexor carpi ulnaris, medial half of flexor digitorum profundus, and muscles of the hand (except thenar muscles and lateral two lumbricals of hand). |
| **Sensory function** | Innervates the anterior and posterior surfaces of the medial index and half of the medial finger palm. |
| **Clinical sign: high lesion** | Injury is proximal to the elbow. Radial extension at the wrist, IP joint flexion, loss of the hypothenar and intrinsic muscles, and clawing at ring and small fingers. |
| **Clinical sign: low lesion** | Injury at level of wrist. Loss of hypothenar and intrinsic muscles, clawing at ring and small fingers, and greater IP flexion deformity. |
| **Treatments** | Passive ROM to avoid PIP flexion contractures and maintain MP flexion and IP extension, splinting, adaptive equipment including built-up handles for ADL tasks as well as modifications/adaptive techniques for loss of sensation. |

## RADIAL NERVE

The radial nerve communicates sensation and motor function through the back of the arm. Numbness, tingling, pain, a burning sensation, as well as deficits with wrist and finger movement can be the result of radial nerve damage.

| | |
|---|---|
| **Nerve root origin** | A peripheral nerve that originates in the brachial plexus and is the terminal continuation of the posterior cord coming from nerve roots C5–T1. |
| **Major branches** | The radial nerve travels anteriorly to the lateral epicondyle of the humerus and divides into two branches. The deep branch is motor based and innervates the muscles in the posterior compartment, and the superficial branch is sensory based and innervates the dorsal hand and fingers. |
| **Motor function** | Innervates the three heads of the triceps brachii and the posterior forearm. |
| **Sensory function** | Innervates the lateral aspect of the arm, the posterior surface of the arm, and the middle of the posterior forearm. |
| **Clinical sign: high lesion** | Forearm pronation, wrist flexion, loss of sensation to the hand, incomplete extension in the wrist and palmar abduction of the thumb. |
| **Clinical sign: low lesion** | Radial wrist extension, deficits and incomplete MP joint extension in the fingers and thumb, sensory loss. |
| **Treatments** | Dynamic splinting, AAROM, modification and adaptive techniques for loss of sensation. |

## SPINE CURVATURES

Lordosis, kyphosis, and scoliosis are all curvatures of the spine. Everyone's spine curves in the neck, upper back, and lower back, creating an S shape for shock absorption, movement, alignment, head support, and balance.

| Condition | Definition |
|---|---|
| Lordosis | Also known as being sway backed. The lower lumbar region of the back is concave, making the buttocks look pronounced. This condition cannot be cured. The patient is placed in a back brace. Therapy treatment includes exercises for strength, ROM, and flexibility. |
| Kyphosis | Also known as being hunch backed. The thoracic region of the back is convex, making the shoulders look rounded and in a constant forward position. This condition cannot be cured. Back braces are worn. Therapy treatment includes exercises for strength, ROM, and flexibility. |
| Scoliosis | A side curvature of the spine. This condition cannot be cured. Back braces are worn. Possible surgery and spinal fusions are indicated. Therapy treatment includes exercises for strength, ROM, and flexibility. |

## COMMON BACK BRACES USED FOR ORTHOPEDIC PATIENTS

Back and neck braces are commonly used after a procedure, injury, or trauma or to treat a spinal disorder or deformity. Therapy treatment will revolve around maintaining back and neck precautions and completing ADLs safely.

- **Corset back brace:** Used for stabilization after spinal fusions, spinal stenosis, laminectomies, and discectomies. Provides support from T9 to S1. Made of rigid plastic and fabric fastened with Velcro with adjustable pieces that can tighten and add more support. Can usually be put on at the edge of the bed when sitting.

- **Clamshell:** Used for stabilization to hold the thoracic spine immobile after spinal fusions, spinal stenosis, laminectomies, discectomies, or spinal cord injury. Made of rigid plastic with Velcro adjustable pieces on the side that can tighten and add more support. There are two separate pieces, and this brace must be applied while the patient is supine in bed using the log-rolling technique.

## COMMON NECK BRACES USED FOR ORTHOPEDIC PATIENTS

Neck braces include the following:

| Brace | Description |
|---|---|
| Miami J or Philadelphia collar | Hard and rigid cervical spine immobilizer. Made of plastic with removable pads. Attached with Velcro. Applied laying supine in bed. Used to restrict neck movement during recovery from fracture or cervical fusion surgery. |
| Soft collar | A flexible and soft brace made of rubber and covered in cotton. Attaches with Velcro. May be applied while sitting. Used to restrict neck movement during recovery from whiplash, fracture, or surgery. |
| Halo | A metal brace that encircles the head with pins screwed into the skull to keep it in place. There are metal rods that connect the halo to a chest piece for stability. Used after a spinal cord injury when the head and neck must remain stable and not move. |
| Sternal occipital mandibular immobilizer | Hard and rigid cervical spine immobilizer. Positions the neck in straight alignment with the spine. Applied laying supine in bed. Used to restrict neck movement during recovery from low cervical and high thoracic fractures or cervical fusion surgery. |

## CP CLASSIFICATIONS

Cerebral palsy (CP) is a neural disorder caused by intracranial lesions.

- **Spastic CP** is caused by damage to the motor cortex and the pyramidal tracts of the brain. This causes rigid muscle tone. It can be spastic diplegia (affecting the legs), spastic hemiplegia (affecting one side of the body), or spastic quadriplegia (affecting all four limbs, the trunk, and face). This is the most common type of CP.
- **Athetoid CP** is also known as dyskinetic CP. It causes abnormal, involuntary movement including fluctuations between hypertonia and hypotonia. It is caused by damage to the basal ganglia and cerebellum. There are categories in this type of CP to classify the type of movement. The most common are dyskinesia (general involuntary movement), dystonia (slow, rotational movement of the extremities and trunk), chorea (random involuntary movements), ataxia (loss of coordination and balance), and rigidity (high tone that inhibits movement).
- **Ataxic CP** affects balance and coordination, causing it to be difficult for the patient to control their movement. It is caused by damage to the cerebellum. This causes difficulty with fine motor precision, mobility, and ADLs due to tremors and random uncontrolled movement.
- **Mixed CP** is the combination of at least two forms of CP. The cause can be damage to one or more areas of the brain including the motor cortex, pyramidal tracts, basal ganglia, and cerebellum. Symptoms can vary from high and low tone to deficits with balance and coordination.

## TYPES OF PALSY

Palsy refers to various types of paralysis throughout the body. The following are the most common types of palsy and how they are addressed in therapy:

| Type of Palsy | Description | Treatment Intervention |
|---|---|---|
| Bell's | Facial paralysis from damage or trauma to the facial nerves. The nerve that controls the facial muscles is swollen, inflamed, or compressed. Symptoms vary from mild weakness to total paralysis. | Protecting the face and eyes from injury including manually blinking, initiation and facilitation of movement exercises for ROM and strengthening of the face, refining movement, modifying ADLs including eating techniques, sensory activity, self-esteem and leisure pursuits, and caregiver education. |
| Cerebral | A neural disorder caused by intracranial lesions that affect the movement of the entire body. | Strengthening, ROM, environmental modifications, seating, ADLs, sensory, cognition training, leisure and hobby pursuits, refining movement, social skills, play skills, and caregiver education. |
| Bulbar | Caused by lower motor neuron lesions in the medulla oblongata and cranial nerves outside the brain stem. Can cause weakness in the arms and legs in addition to facial deficits including swallowing issues; a weak jaw, tongue, and facial muscles; and progressive loss of speech. | Strengthening, ROM, environmental modifications, ADLs, leisure and hobby pursuits, refining movement, sensory activities, social skills, play skills, and caregiver education. |
| Erb's | Also known as birth palsy. It is caused by paralysis of the arm caused by injury to the brachial plexus at the upper trunk of C5–C6. It can cause weakness and sensation loss in the affected arm or partial or total paralysis of the arm. | Splinting, ROM, environmental modifications, ADLs, leisure and hobby pursuits, refining movement, sensory activities, social skills, play skills, and caregiver education. |

## HYPERTONIA VS. HYPOTONIA

**Hypertonia** is increased muscle tone with lack of flexibility caused by damage or injury to the brain or spinal cord. Patients who are hypertonic often have stiff and rigid movements and will show deficits with basic mobility, transfers, and ADLs. **Hypotonia** is decreased muscle tone and too much flexibility and is caused by damage to the central nervous system, muscle disorders, and genetic disorders. Patients who are hypotonic are often referred to as "floppy" or having low muscle tone. Treatment for both conditions will include strengthening and stretching exercises, ADL modifications, fine motor tasks, transfer training, balance tasks, orthotics and splinting, postural stability, adaptive equipment, and modified leisure pursuits.

## REFLEX SYMPATHETIC DYSTROPHY

**Reflex sympathetic dystrophy** is a form of complex regional pain syndrome. This is a chronic condition with symptoms that include severe, burning pain in the extremities and extreme sensitivity to touch. It also causes pathological changes of the bones, joints, and skin as well as edema and excessive sweating. It can be categorized as Type 1, which is not caused by a nerve injury, or Type 2, which is caused by a distinct nerve injury. The symptoms can come from trauma or nerve damage, but they often occur without any identified previous injury or illness. Every aspect of the patient's life is affected by pain, and movement and independence are difficult. In treatment, psychosocial aspects are key, monitoring for depression, coping techniques, and encouraging leisure pursuits and hobbies. Desensitization techniques can be helpful as are joint compression ROM, strengthening, ADLs, and stress loading protocols for the affected joints that involve scrubbing and carrying techniques.

## SEIZURES

A **seizure** is a chemical change in the nerve cells causing a surge of electricity in the brain that inhibits brain cells from sending proper messages to the rest of the body. Seizures can present differently in each person. the six types of seizures are as follows:

- **Atonic seizures**, lasting for fewer than 15 seconds, are also known as drop seizures because the patient will fall immediately to the ground. There is a loss of muscle strength, and the patient will feel tired but recover quickly.
- **Clonic seizures** are rare, cause repeated flexing and extending of the muscles in a jerking movement, and may last up to 2 minutes. It is difficult to tell clonic and myoclonic seizures apart at times. Clonic seizures affect both sides of the brain at once. The patient will feel tired but recover quickly.
- **Myoclonic seizures** are considered as general seizures with quick muscle jerking, and they can last upwards of 30 minutes. There is minimal consciousness, recovery is slow, and the patient may present as sleepy and confused.
- **Petit mal/absence seizures** last for fewer than 15 seconds, and they may not be noticeable. There may be a loss of conscience, and it may look like the patient is staring blankly into space. There may be a loss of movement without falling and a quick recovery.
- **Grand mal/tonic-clonic seizures** are when patient loses consciousness, the muscles stiffen, and there may be convulsions. The patient may bite his or her tongue and may present as sleepy and confused. These seizures may last up to 5 minutes, they will cause falling, and recovery is slow.
- **Tonic seizures** are when there is increased extensor tone in the muscles and all limbs. These seizures last fewer than 30 seconds, will cause a loss of balance and falling, and recovery is slow. The patient may present as sleepy and confused.

## SAFE PATIENT HANDLING

Back injuries are common in healthcare workers most often because of the frequency of transferring and mobilizing patients. Injuries are frequent when lifting or mobilizing alone, mobilizing and lifting an uncooperative or confused patient, and when moving a patient that can't support their own weight. Basic guidelines for safe patient handling are to never lift more than you can comfortably handle, keep a wide base of support, and bend your knees while lifting with your legs and not your back. Gait belts are used in most facilities and are placed around a patient's waist for a more secure grasp when moving and ambulating.

### STAND/SQUAT PIVOT TRANSFER

Position the patient so that his stronger side is closest to the surface that he is transferring onto, and ensure that the destination and the current surfaces are locked in place. Explain what is happening to the patient. Have the patient slide his hips forward, one at a time to get to the front edge of the surface. Place the gait belt. Use your knees to block the patient so that he doesn't slip off the surface. Have him shift his body weight forward like he is going to hug you, and have him place his hands around your waist or elbows while you hold the gait belt. Give the patient a count or cue to stand. When he stands (fully upright or in a squat), block his legs by placing your feet and knees outside of the patient's feet and knees to avoid buckling. Pivot your feet toward the transfer surface, rotating the patient over the destination surface. Hold onto the patient as you help him lower himself to the destination surface.

## USING A TRANSFER/SLIDE BOARD

A **slide board** is a long piece of plastic or wood that is used to transfer a person who has good trunk control and arm strength but is non-weight-bearing. When the patient is sitting, make sure that the wheels on both pieces of equipment are locked. Explain what is happening to the patient, and place the gait belt. Have the patient lean to the side opposite of the transfer and place one-quarter of the slide board under the buttock with the rest of the board over the area of the gap between the two surfaces with the opposite end resting on the destination surface. Make sure that the patient's feet are on the floor and stand close blocking his knees so he won't slide off the board. Have the patient slide his buttock across the board toward the destination surface using a small, short pushing movement while keeping the hands flat and the feet on the floor for balance. When the patient has reached his destination surface, have him lean toward the surface he just arrived on to remove and pull the board out from under his buttock.

## COMPLETING A LATERAL TRANSFER

This is a transfer of a patient between two horizontal surfaces such as a bed to a stretcher, geri chair, or gurney. Make sure that the wheels on both pieces of equipment are locked. A minimum of two people is required to complete a lateral transfer. Explain what is happening to the patient and what they need to do. Raise the bed to a safe working height, and lower the head of the bed and the side rails. Roll the patient over, and place the slider board halfway under the patient making sure there is a sheet between the patient and the board. The person on the far side of the bed will push the patient to arm's length across the surface, and the person on the far side will use his body weight to bring the patient with them using the sheet to the new surface.

## COMPLETING A DEPENDENT OR MECHANICAL LIFT

A **dependent lift** is the use of a mechanical lift machine to move a patient that is immobile and unable to bear weight. **Mechanical lifts** can be electric or manual. Two staff are needed for a mechanical lift. Make sure that the patient understands what is happening. When the patient is lying supine in bed, have her roll side to side to place the sling underneath her securely. Position the lift so that the legs of it are opened wide and under the bed for increased stabilization. Raise the bed up and attach the loops on the sling to the hooks of the mechanical lift. Raise the patient up until the sling clears the bed. As the lift is moved away from the bed, one person should be supporting the base and moving the lift while the other is supporting the patient's head and directing the sling. When the patient is positioned over the chair, the person who was stabilizing the sling needs to move behind the chair and stabilize the chair and pull the sling toward the back of the chair to position the patient while the other person lowers the lift arm. The loops are removed from the lift hooks, but the sling remains under the patient for ease when transferring back to the bed.

## DEVICES USED IN THERAPY

When a patient has been in bed for an extended amount of time due to injury and illness, they often have blood pressure issues and become orthostatic and have difficulty returning to activity including sitting. Using a tilt table, thrombo-embolic deterrent (TED) hose, and abdominal binders can help maintain stable pressure and prevent syncope when working on activity and upright tolerance.

- **Tilt table**: This is a special bed or table with special multiple safety belts and a footrest that can be slowly raised into standing to address activity tolerance and monitor blood pressure with change of position.
- **TED hose**: This is a compression garment worn on the legs by nonambulatory patients who are at a high risk for blood clots. TED hose has compression levels of 20 mm Hg or less.
- **Abdominal binder**: This is an elastic compression band that is wide and attaches with Velcro. It applies compression to the abdomen and can help prevent blood pooling seen with an orthostatic blood pressure drop. It is also used for pain relief, to keep drains in place after abdominal surgery, and to support deep diaphragmatic breathing.

## AREAS AND ITEMS TO REVIEW FOR ACCESSIBILITY IN HOME EVALUATIONS

A home evaluation is provided to a patient prior to discharge home from a facility. It is often done partnered with a physical therapist, and the patient is always present during the evaluation so that they can demonstrate how they can complete daily tasks safely and independently. The goal is to assess the patient's mobility and independence in the natural environment and how the living setup either supports or limits the patient's functioning and lifestyle. The general, most basic features and areas you would inspect are as follows:

- **Entry into the home**: stairs, handrails, ramps, lights, safety strips, and safety concerns
- **General home features**: alarm systems, peephole availability and location on doors, fire and carbon monoxide alarms, phones/land-line locations, extension cord placement, fire extinguishers, thermostats, water shutoff, breaker boxes, electrical outlets, evacuation plans, placement of furniture for maneuverability, flooring surfaces, lighting, locks and door handles, overall doorway openings, and water heater temperature.

### KITCHEN, BEDROOM, AND BATHROOM

The home safety evaluation is designed to increase independence, functional performance, and safety while attempting to decrease the chance of injury in the home. Based on these findings, the therapist can create a plan for short- or long-term home safety and accessibility. The three key areas to assess for safety and function are the bathroom, bedroom, and kitchen.

- **Kitchen**: Assess the cook top (gas/electric, knob placement, and adaptive devices), counter space and cabinets (height, depth, width, locations, shapes, type, and handles), fire extinguishers, oven and microwave height/placement, refrigerator type/height/placement, sink (depth/width/height/faucet/shape/disposal location), garbage accessibility including type of can, flooring, pantry accessibility, accessibility of small appliances (toaster, blender), and throw rugs.
- **Bedroom**: Assess the bed size, transfer equipment, distance to the bathroom, location, closet size and accessibility to clothing, furniture placement, throw rugs and flooring, light sources, and outlets.
- **Bathroom**: Can they get in the room with their device (walker/wheelchair)? Do the drains work? Assess the lighting, plug locations, grab bars, turning radius, toilet height, tub versus shower, shower seat, nonslip flooring, throw rugs, shower heads, access to medicine cabinet, and faucet and handle accessibility.

## ADL Modifications
### Dressing and Grooming

Clothing is where many people express their individuality and make a statement. Being unable to dress independently or wear the things you want to wear can have a significant impact on self-esteem and confidence. The following are the most common items that are used to assist with dressing:

- **Button hook**: Allows for one-handed buttoning when there are fine motor, vision, and dexterity deficits.
- **Elastic laces**: These will turn any pair of lace-up shoes into slip-ons. Works well for patients that are obese or unable to bend over or for those that have fine motor, vision, and dexterity deficits.
- **Sock aid**: This allows the patient to don socks without bending over or breaking hip precautions. There are also sturdier devices that will help the patient to don compression stockings.
- **Dressing stick**: This will assist a patient with ROM deficits, difficulty bending, or the use of only one arm to dress independently.
- **Long-handled shoehorn**: This is a long plastic wand with a shoehorn attached so that the patient can get their shoe on without bending over.
- **Reacher**: The jack of all trades piece of equipment. This will allow a patient with limited ROM get clothes out of the closet or out of drawers, pick up items that are dropped without bending over, and don pants while maintaining hip precautions.

### Eating

It is important for patients to return to activities that are essential for taking caring of themselves and maintaining independence. One of the most basic life skills is preparing and eating simple meals. The following pieces of equipment are the most common adaptive kitchen items used to assist a patient in completing these tasks independently:

- **Modified knives/Rocker knives**: Used for one-handed cutting. Works well for patients post stroke or for those with Parkinson's, multiple sclerosis, muscle weakness, or arthritis.
- **Plate guards**: Used to keep food on the plate and to scoop food onto a utensil. Food can be pushed by a utensil against the ridge along the edge of the plate.
- **Angled/Swivel utensils**: Keep food in the same position while the handle of the utensil moves.
- **Weighted and built-up handle utensils**: Help stabilize against tremors or uncontrolled movements that cause food to drop from the utensil before it travels to the mouth, and they require less fine motor control and a larger surface area for a weaker grip.
- **Sippy cups/Cups with handles and use of lids and straws**: Allow liquid to not spill due to tremors or uncontrolled movements; there is a larger surface area to hold onto including a handle to hold the fingers in place.

## KITCHEN

The following are the most common adaptive kitchen items and modifications used to assist a patient in completing these tasks independently:

- **Dycem**: A nonslip product that comes in rolls. It is used on chairs for extra traction, to assist with grip opening jars and bottles, as a placemat to keep plates in one place and stable, and under kitchen chair legs to keep the chair from scooting. Works well for anyone with a poor grip.
- **Stove knob modifications**: pieces are put over the standard knobs to provide a greater surface area.
- Using a chair to sit on while working at the stove or completing meal prep while seated at a table.

## TOILETING HYGIENE AND PERI CARE

The following are the most common pieces of adaptive equipment and devices used in toileting hygiene and peri care:

- **Commode/Three-in-one commode**: This has a raised seat, an armrest on both sides of the chair, and a removable bucket, so it can work as a shower chair, a bedside commode, or over the toilet in the bathroom to make getting on and off the toilet easier.
- **Self-wipe toilet aid**: This is a long plastic wand with a bent and flexible tip to hold toilet paper for peri care for patients that can't reach to get themselves clean.
- **Long-handle sponge/brush**: This is a long plastic wand with a sponge or brush attached so that the patient can wash their back, groin, or feet without bending over, and they can also brush their hair without raising their arms too far overhead.

Loss of personal care independence, specifically in the bathroom, is one of the most devastating things that your patient may face. What was once private and easy now often requires a multiple-person assist.

- **Grab bars**: These can be permanently attached or attached via suction cups. They are to assist with stability getting in and out of the shower and on/off the toilet.
- **Handheld shower wand**: This allows the freedom to sit during bathing, aiming the wand toward the area that needs to be rinsed.
- **Shower seat**: A plastic chair or built-in fold-down seat with or without a back, with rubber tips on the bottom to prevent sliding.
- **Tub bench**: This is a seating device in the tub that extends to the outside of the tub. The extended part of the bench is where the patient sits and slides across into the tub without having to step over the tub. The patient will lean back and lift her legs over the side of the tub.

## UNIVERSAL DESIGN AND REASONABLE ACCOMMODATIONS

**Universal design** is the process of creating products that are accessible to all people with a wide range of abilities and disabilities without discrimination based on age, size, ability, or disability. The overall goal is to increase functional performance and decrease the complexity of the design. The Americans with Disabilities Act (ADA) prohibits employment discrimination on the basis of workers' disabilities, and it also requires employers to provide reasonable accommodations for employees with disabilities to do their jobs. **Reasonable accommodations** can include changing work schedule hours, modifying test and training manuals, modifying workstations, providing adaptive equipment, and providing mentors and assistants for training. Again, under the ADA, fair housing laws require a housing provider to make reasonable accommodations in the home. This can include closer parking spots, allowing service animals without extra fees, providing ramps or elevator access, widening doors, and changing knobs and door handles.

## DME

**Durable medical equipment** (DME) are items that serve a medical purpose, are prescribed by a physician, are reusable, and can sustain repeated use over a significant amount of time. Medicare will cover DME if the equipment is durable, designed to help a medical condition, used in the home, and are likely to last for three years or more. Durable medical devices can be mobility aids; orthotics; and ADL equipment including commodes, hospital beds, oxygen equipment, and insulin pumps. Mobility aids are specialized items that help increase independence and mobility. They can be canes, walkers, rollators, crutches, ramps, scooters, and lift chairs.

### HIGH- AND LOW-TECH ASSISTIVE DEVICES AND HUMAN INTERFACE ASSESSMENT MODEL

**Assistive technology devices** are items or pieces of equipment that are purchased commercially and can be modified and customized as needed in order to increase or improve functional performance for individuals with disabilities. **High-tech assistive devices** are generally more expensive items with electronic components and that will likely require training to learn how to use them. A **low-tech assistive device** is a lower cost item that will be easy to use and not have complicated mechanical features. The **Human Interface Assessment model** examines client skills in four areas (motor, process, communication, and activity demands) in order to understand the strengths and challenges that the patient faces daily so that appropriate assistive technology can be recommended.

| Low-Tech Assistive Devices | High-Tech Assistive Devices |
|---|---|
| Pen grips, handheld magnifiers, canes, walkers, reachers, audiobooks, large-print text, visual schedulers, adaptive pens and paper, slant boards, highlighters, Post-its, fidget toys, and manipulatives. | Computers with specialized software, voice recognition, wireless, and Bluetooth technology. Power chairs and scooters, scanning and eye-gaze items, touch screens, optical character recognition, text-to-speech devices, screen enlargement, trackballs, tongue-touch keypads, Sip-N-Puff technology, alerting devices, and smart boards. |

## CONSIDERATIONS WHEN DECIDING BETWEEN A POWER VERSUS STANDARD WHEELCHAIR

There are many determinations in deciding if a manual or power chair is a better option for your patient.

| | Pros | Cons |
|---|---|---|
| **Manual chairs** | Less expensive, easy to transport, folds up compactly, does not need to be charged, maneuvers in small areas, parts can be replaced quickly, can be picked up with the patient in the chair to get upstairs if a ramp is unavailable, and easily covered by insurance. | Need good UE strength to propel independently; can cause repetitive movement injury with long-term use; difficult to maneuver over anything but a flat, even surface; and difficult to use chair locks/brakes. |
| **Power chairs** | Don't need to propel with arms so there is less chance of fatigue, more options for pressure relief and positioning, can be driven with little effort (joystick/sip-blow control), works on any terrain, sturdier, don't require chair brakes, and more independence in the community for long-distance mobility (going to the grocery store alone). | Very expensive to purchase, may be difficult to get parts and repair, transport would require a lift on a car to carry it, needs to be charged, battery is costly to replace, can cause damage to the door and walls when turning and moving about the space, and need significant documentation to get insurance to cover. |

## WHEELCHAIR FITTING

Every patient will have very specific needs for a wheelchair and seating system based on the type and level of injury, skin integrity, and mobility. A wheelchair that does not fit well can cause pressure ulcers and may lead to posture and balance issues and difficulty mobilizing the chair independently. It is important to remember the 90-90-90 rule for posture when fitting the chair. This rule states that good posture requires a 90° bend at the hips, knees, and ankles. According to the ADA, a standard manual wheelchair's dimensions are as follows: eye level, 43–51 inches; lap height, 27 inches; armrest height, 30 inches; and seat height, 19 inches. The following are the measurements needed when fitting a patient for a chair in addition to listing their height, weight, and diagnosis:

- hip width (chair width)
- hip to popliteal fossa (chair depth)
- shoulder width (chair width)
- chest width and depth (width of the chair back)
- knee to heel (leg rest length and set to floor height)
- inferior angle of the scapula (chair back height)
- top of the shoulder (height of the back of the chair)
- top of the head (to determine the headrest height)
- elbow to mat (armrest height)
- elbow to wrist and fingertip (length of the armrest)
- foot length and width (size and length of the foot plates).

## DIFFERENT SEATING SYSTEMS USED IN WHEELCHAIRS

Seating systems in wheelchairs are not just about comfort. They are specifically designed for positioning needs, pressure relief, and posture. Different diagnoses and amounts of time in a chair will dictate what the best choice for a seating system is. There are three types of cushions available: gel, air, and foam.

| Type | Details |
|---|---|
| Gel | Expensive option that offers positioning and pressure relief including off-loading areas of concern. Very stable, but cumbersome. |
| Air | Can be expensive depending on the brand. Good pressure relief, and the firmness can be adjusted easily. It is the least stable surface and can develop leaks. |
| Foam | It is the most basic and inexpensive option, being firm and stable but not conducive to pressure relief. |

## POSITIONING DEVICES

A **positioning device** is something that is used in order to increase and improve independence in functional activity in the least restrictive way and potentially improve occupational performance. The following is a list of how some are used:

- **Wheelchair arm troughs**: Used to increase postural control and support a flaccid or nonfunctional arm.
- **Bolsters**: Used to provide support under a joint during therapeutic exercises or for seated positioning during activity.
- **Wedges**: Used to create proper pelvic tilt in seated activity or use in supine exercise for patients that can't lay completely flat.
- **Lap trays**: Used to prevent the patient from slipping out of the chair during tasks and to promote proper posture. These are never to be used as restraints!
- **Pillows**: Used in positioning in the bed in order to maintain postural alignment; position in side-lying; and to prevent bedsores, float heels, and prevent foot drop.
- **Lap buddies**: Used for proper pelvis alignment in sitting and for increasing postural control. They are also used a gentle reminder to impulsive patients to not get out of a wheelchair without help. They are never to be used as restraints!
- **Clip Seatbelt**: Used to prevent sacral sliding and increase seated mobility and function in a wheelchair. This is never to be used as a restraint!
- **Leg rests**: Used to keep the 90-90-90 required for proper and functional posture.
- **Cushion**: Used to address posture and pressure relief and can address pelvic tilt concerns.

## DRIVER REHABILITATION AND OPTIONS FOR VEHICLE ADAPTATIONS

Driver rehabilitation is an emerging practice area. OTs may seek specialized training in order to provide this type of intervention. Evaluations are in two parts, with the first part being clinic based and the second part involving actually driving. The purpose is to evaluate the patient's physical, visual, and mental abilities required to safely operate a motor vehicle. The testing and activities focus on visual acuity skills, reaction time, and decision making. The therapist will work with the physician to make recommendations about the strategies, specialized equipment, and training needed in order to maintain independence with driving. The following is a list of vehicle adaptation that are commonly used:

- **Driving controls:** push-button start, button gear shifts, modified hand brake, modified pedals, steering wheel knobs and encasements for better grip and a wider steering wheel, and larger rearview mirrors
- **Accessibility:** pivot boards for the seat, seatbelt modifications and extensions, and ramps for wheelchair access.

# Competency and Practice Management

## RHUMBA AND SMART

Every therapist develops their own style of documentation throughout their careers. Goal writing can be tricky and does take practice. As an OT, your goals need to be functional and occupational-based in addition to basic ROM, strengthening, and mobility goals. There are two common acronyms that will help you write your goals correctly: SMART and RHUMBA.

S = Significant
M = Measurable
A = Achievable
R = Relatable
T = Time Based

R = Relevant
H = How long
U = Understandable
M = Measurable
B = Behavioral
A = Achievable

Examples of goals:

- Patient will maintain static standing balance with feet shoulder-width apart and stand-by assist (SBA) to improve safety in the standing position for functional mobility and ADLs 80% of the time within 6 weeks.
- Patient will demonstrate improved endurance and strength for postural control and UE function for sink-side standing grooming activities by maintaining position for 4 minutes with no verbal cues and without the use of a device five times in 3 weeks.

## OCCUPATIONAL THERAPY MANAGER ROLE

The role of an occupational therapy manager can be different depending on the setting. In most cases, in addition to maintaining an active caseload, the job is to provide management and administration of all aspects of rehabilitation services in the facility. The job description will likely contain the following aspects:

- maintaining a clinical caseload with 20%–30% productivity
- responsible for recruiting, retaining, and training rehab staff
- promoting positive department and employee relations with open communication and problem solving
- responsible for conducting performance appraisals, hiring, firing, and discipline issues of all rehabilitative staff
- promoting ethics within the program and making sure that state regulations are being met per the OT/PT/SLP national organizations
- monitors and assists with personnel and compliance issues including credentials, corrective actions, and improvement plans
- assures that all program standards are met (Commission on Accreditation of Rehabilitation Facilities [CARF]/Joint Commission on Accreditation of Healthcare Organizations [JCAHO])
- develop strategies and programming to increase facility revenue

114

- lead efforts to build caseloads within the facility
- program development
- marketing in the community on behalf of facility to increase awareness of the therapy program

## ADMINISTRATORS VS. MANAGERS

Throughout your career as an OT, your role will likely change from that of a patient care therapist into more managerial roles such as manager, supervisor, and even administrator. The variations of each position and productivity standards will vary based on the setting, and the following is a list of the most general responsibilities:

- **Administrator**
  - responsible for overseeing daily operations
  - may need special certifications based on the state and organization (assisted living administrator license)
  - ensuring federal and state compliance is being met
  - will often be involved in community committees and boards in order to help promote and maintain the reputation of the facility or organization
  - delegate many tasks for daily operation
- **Manager**
  - mentor and supervisor for therapists in their department (PT, OT, and speech-language pathology [SLP])
  - scheduling
  - payroll
  - compliance with Medicare and insurance standards
  - often acts as a buffer between therapists and administration
  - interviews therapy staff for recruiting/hiring/firing staff

## LEAD THERAPISTS VS. SUPERVISORS

Throughout your career as an OT, your role will likely change from that of a patient care therapist into more managerial roles such as manager, supervisor, and even administrator. The variations of each position and productivity standards will vary based on the setting, and the following is a list of the most general responsibilities:

- **Lead Therapist**
  - helps set the tone and culture for the rehabilitation department
  - participates in new staff hiring
  - ensures that therapy staff completes required documentation
  - develops programming
  - performs competency assessments and staff development opportunities
- **Supervisor**
  - oversees day-to-day operations of the department
  - empowers and mentors the staff
  - participates in the hiring/firing of staff

## OTPF

The **Occupational Therapy Practice Framework (OTPF)** is an official document of the **American Occupational Therapy Association (AOTA)**. Its purpose is to define the role and the core concepts of OTs in the domain and process. The domain is explained as occupations, performance patterns and skills, client factors and contexts, and environments. The process is considered to be the service delivery models, clinical reasoning, therapeutic use of self, activity analysis, evaluation, intervention, and determining outcomes. The goal of the domain is to support participation and engagement in a person's life through occupational performance. The goal of the process is to evaluate the patient's occupational needs, problems, and concerns.

## GUIDELINES FOR DOCUMENTATION ESTABLISHED BY AOTA

AOTA has established documentations guidelines based on the OTPF. Occupational therapy documentation always needs to record the therapist's activities in the areas of evaluation, intervention, and outcomes. There are four areas that need to be established in documentation:

1. Establish the rationale for occupational therapy and how and why services will impact and affect the patient's outcome.
2. Documentation will establish and reflect the judgment and clinical reasoning of the therapist.
3. Communicate and establish clinical information with an occupational therapy perspective.
4. Create a chronological perspective of the treatment, services, and outcomes of the patient's therapy sessions and process.

## PRESENT IN ALL DOCUMENTATION

Within the areas of evaluation, intervention, and outcome documentation, the following always need to be present in all documentation:

- Client's full name and record number.
- Date and type of occupational therapy contact (evaluation, reevaluation, treatment, or discharge).
- Identification of agency and department name (for example, Memorial Hospital, inpatient therapy services).
- OT signature with professional credentials.
- Cosign space on documentation written by students and occupational therapy assistants.
- Acceptable terminology defined within the boundaries of the setting. Most facilities have an issued document with their approved abbreviations.
- In written documents, errors are corrected by drawing a single line through an error and by initialing the correction (correction tape or fluid and erasures are not acceptable in any legal medical record).

## WHAT MAKES FOR GOOD DOCUMENTATION

Documentation is the primary communication tool among healthcare providers and to justify services for reimbursement. It is also a legal document that must withstand scrutiny even years later. Good documentation is accurate and objective and clearly identifies the intervention to the patient and the patient's response. Most documentation is now electronic, but it is always possible that you may have to document on paper. Documentation needs to be legible, and only facility-approved and -recognized abbreviations should be used. Most seasoned therapists will tell all new providers, "If you don't write it down, it didn't happen." If any portion of the treatment is not documented and identified, it leaves the door open for doubt about the patient's care and could be a potential liability if the patient's case is ever taken to court. Documenting with the thought that someday you may need to justify and defend your service in a court of law is the best course of action for protecting yourself now and in the future.

## DOCUMENTING SKILLED SERVICES, MEDICAL APPROPRIATENESS, AND A MODIFIED PLAN OF CARE

Skilled and detailed documentation is essential for reimbursement and will determine if services will be covered and paid to a provider.

- Detailed description of the skilled services provided (accuracy of task performance, number and type of cuing needed, speed of response or action with a task, level of independence, frequency and number of attempts)
  - The therapist provides verbal cues with Min A for seated balance at the EOB to instruct the patient in a compensatory strategy in order to use one-handed techniques for donning socks and shoes and for putting the appropriate shoe on the correct foot. These specific instructions and cues provided to the patient are important to the patient learning the task and to further independence in ADLs.
- Why treatment is medically appropriate
  - Patient with significant balance issues s/p stroke per his score of 1 on the four-stage balance test. The patient must demonstrate lower body dressing skills with SBA while maintaining standing balance in order to return home to his assisted living facility.
- The decision-making process that caused you to modify treatment and POC
  - The patient continues to have difficulty with getting from supine to sitting when transitioning out of bed independently. The patient has been successful on two of five attempts using a bed rail to get to the EOB. New goal added on 9/24/18 for strength in crossing midline to address reaching for the bed rail to increase independence with bed mobility.

## DOCUMENTING USING TECHNICAL KNOWLEDGE, A PATIENT'S RESPONSE TO SERVICES, AND PROGRESS TOWARD GOALS

Once the basics of note writing are learned, documentation becomes second nature for a therapist and a rhythm of common phrases will emerge. As long as you cover the basics, note writing is an individual process, and it becomes easy to detail even the smallest aspects of progress.

- Using terminology that reflects your technical knowledge
  - Pt is 6 weeks s/p carpal tunnel repair and continues to have moderate pitting edema in the left wrist and hand. Guarding with AROM due to pain. Soft-tissue limitations for PROM/AAROM. Able to use a gross grasp and pinch with the left hand. Fine motor skills are still significantly limited by strength.
- Assessment of the patient's response to the services
  - After demonstration of cuing techniques for patient's HEP, caregiver was able to use similar cuing techniques on the next three exercises for carryover at home.
- Progress toward the treatment goals
  - Pt is now using compensatory strategies (picture board) for orientation to time and to express needs to reduce agitation with 50% accuracy when cued by the staff and family.

## DOCUMENTING MEDICAL NECESSITY

In order to document medical necessity, the chart must detail specifics about the reasons that diagnostic and treatment decisions were made for the patient. Because healthcare has turned into a fee-for-service delivery program, which means that you get paid for what you do, documentation is key for reimbursement and proving medical necessity can make the difference between being paid or not being paid. A treatment being deemed not medically necessary is one of the top reasons for a claim to be denied.

## DOCUMENTING COMPLEXITY OF TREATMENT, LEVEL OF ASSISTANCE, AND OBJECTIVE MEASURES

The following are examples of documenting complexity of treatment, level of assistance, and objective measures:

- **Complexity of the treatment:** To address word memory and cognitive skills, the patient names four items within a category. A limit of 15 seconds makes the activity more complex than during previous sessions.
- **Objective measures:** The four-stage balance test is a test for static balance. There are four positions in the test: (1) parallel stance, (2) semitandem stance, (3) tandem (heel-toe) stance, and (4) one-legged stance. Patients aged 65 years or older who do not progress to the tandem (heel-toe) stance or cannot hold this stance for at least 10 seconds are at an increased risk of falling.
- **Current level of assistance needed for functional tasks:** A patient requires moderate verbal cues and Min A in order to manage clothing and complete peri care in toiling activities.

## NBCOT STANDARDS OF PRACTICE

The **NBCOT Professional Practice Standards for OTR** is a document established by NBCOT to define and explain what occupational therapy practitioners should and should not do when providing services to a patient. These are the minimum requirements that a therapist is accountable for when providing services. There is a set of practice standards for registered occupational therapists (OTRs) and occupational therapy assistants (OTAs). The standards of practice have four categories:

1. Practice domains
   a. Acquire information regarding factors that influence occupational performance throughout the occupational therapy process.
   b. Formulate conclusions regarding client needs and priorities to develop and monitor an intervention plan throughout the occupational therapy process.
   c. Select interventions for managing a client-centered plan throughout the occupational therapy process.
   d. Manage and direct occupational therapy services to promote quality in practice.
2. Code of professional conduct
3. Supervision
   a. Direct and indirect supervision based on state rules and regulations
4. Documentation
   a. Rules and regulations about what is required and needed when documenting care.

## NBCOT CODE OF CONDUCT

The **code of conduct** is a document established by the National Board of Certification of Occupational Therapy (NBCOT) to define and explain the standards of personal and professional conduct expected by OTs and required for licensing and certification. It is expected that all occupational therapy practitioners behave with moral and ethical standards. There are nine principles in the code of conduct.

1. Certificants shall provide accurate, truthful, and timely representations to NBCOT.
2. Certificants who are the subject of a qualifications and compliance review shall cooperate with NBCOT concerning investigations and requests for relevant information.
3. Certificants shall be accurate, truthful, and complete in any and all communications, direct or indirect, with any client, employer, regulatory agency, or other parties as they relate to their professional work, education, professional credentials, research, and contributions to the field of occupational therapy.
4. Certificants shall comply with state and/or federal laws, regulations, and statutes governing the practice of occupational therapy.
5. Certificants shall not have been convicted of a serious crime.
6. Certificants shall not engage in behavior or conduct, lawful or otherwise, that causes them to be, or reasonably perceived to be, a threat or potential threat to the health, well-being, or safety of recipients or potential recipients of occupational therapy services.
7. Certificants shall not engage in the practice of occupational therapy while one's ability to practice is impaired due to chemical (i.e., legal and/or illegal) drug or alcohol abuse.
8. Certificants shall not electronically post personal health information or anything, including photos, that may reveal a patient's/client's identity or personal or therapeutic relationship.
9. Certificants shall not misuse NBCOT's intellectual property, certification marks, logos, or other copyrighted materials.

## NBCOT's Disciplinary Action Summary

A violation against the code of conduct is a serious issue that can lead to the termination of your license and ability to practice as an OT. A complaint can be made via the NBCOT website, and a form will be filled out. A complaint cannot be made anonymously because an accused therapist has the right to know who is making an accusation. Once complaints are made, investigations are launched that can take 6–9 months or longer to investigate thoroughly. Sanctions can include the following:

- **Ineligibility for certification** - not being able to sit for the exam at any time
- **Reprimand** - a formal written letter of disapproval, which is attached to the therapist's file, but is not made public
- **Censure** - formal written letter of disapproval that is made public
- **Probation** - maintaining certification is subject to conditions: monitoring, education, or counseling
- **Suspension** - loss of certification for a specific amount of time before you can apply for reinstatement
- **Revocation** - permanent loss of certification and you can no longer practice or identify as a therapist

## License and Certification Requirements

In order to become a licensed OT, a person must have graduated from an accredited school of occupational therapy's program and completed fieldwork, pass the NBCOT licensing exam, and be licensed in the state that they will practice in. State certification requirements can vary from state to state, but they will likely include proof of graduation from an accredited OT program, proof of passing the NBCOT exam, reference letters, and possibly a jurisprudence or specialized test in addition to whatever fees are required by that state. If you are currently licensed in a state and apply for a license in another state, often just proof of an active license in another state is all you will need.

119

## CONTINUING EDUCATION REQUIREMENTS FOR MAINTAINING A LICENSE

Continuing education is required in order to maintain your license both at the national level with NBCOT and at the state level, which will vary based on the state you practice in. The NBCOT certification requires 36 hours during the 3-year renewal cycle. States will require anywhere from 12 to 36 units each renewal cycle. You should always determine if the class provider is someone who is an authorized provider of continuing education units (CEUs)/professional development units (PDUs) by AOTA before you register for a class so that you can be sure the time and money spent will apply to maintain your license. **PDUs** are earned for each contact hour spent in a class setting. A **CEU** is equal to 10 contact hours. Continuing education hours can come in more forms besides taking in-person and online classes. You can also earn hours by writing papers, conducting research, taking fieldwork students, performing volunteer work, presenting information at conferences, publishing, and providing training and in-services.

## SUPERVISION REQUIREMENTS FOR COTAS

Supervision of certified occupational therapy assistants (COTAs) will vary from state to state, and AOTA has a complete list of each state's supervision requirements on its webpage. The COTA is practicing under your license, and it is up to you to determine the level of supervision that you are comfortable with. Generally speaking, OTs are not allowed to supervise more than three COTAs and two technicians at one time without written authorization from their state board. Each facility will handle how an OT will sign off on notes and supervise differently based on setting and therapist experience. The most basic categories of supervision are as follows:

- **Direct supervision**: The supervising OT is in the immediate area of the occupational therapy assistant while performing supportive services.
- **Close supervision**: The supervising OT provides initial direction to the occupational therapy assistant and daily contact while on the premises at least 50% of the direct patient care hours per month.
- **General supervision**: The supervising OT has face-to-face contact with the occupational therapy assistant at least once every 14–30 calendar days, with the supervising OT available by telephone, electronic, or written communication.

## LIFE-THREATENING SITUATIONS AND THE BASIC TYPES OF CODES IN A MEDICAL SETTING

Every medical facility is different and has their own internal rules for how to handle an emergent situation. Most institutions use colors (code red, code blue) to identify specific types of emergencies. In the event of an emergency, the staff are trained to recognize and respond appropriately to these announcements including moving patients, checking rooms, and monitoring doors. These are the basic code colors and definitions used, but may vary between facilities.

| Code | Definition |
| --- | --- |
| Blue | Cardiac emergency (heart or respiration) |
| Red | Fire |
| Green | Combative person |
| Pink | Child or infant abduction |
| Orange | Hazardous spills |
| Silver | Weapon or hostage situation |
| Purple | Internal triage (computer network down for documenting and medication, major plumbing problems/flood, and power or telephone outage) |
| Yellow | External triage (mass casualties; severe weather; massive power outages and nuclear, biological, or chemical accidents). |
| Black | Active shooter/terrorist attack. |
| Rapid Response | Medical team needed at bedside; not at the point of needing a code team, but the patient is declining fast and needs intervention before a code blue is needed. |
| All clear | Announced when the emergency is over usually stated over the loudspeaker 3× (code green, all clear). |

## RISK MANAGEMENT TECHNIQUES IN HEALTHCARE

Risk management is the ability to reduce financial liability and exposure in preventing harm to patients and reducing medical malpractice. Most facilities will have a risk management officer that will help to find and improve areas of concern before a sentinel event can occur. According to The Joint Commission, a sentinel event is an "unanticipated event in a healthcare setting resulting in death or serious physical or psychological injury to a patient or patients, not related to the natural course of the patient's illness." The best proactive approach is for risk managers to perform risk assessments and identify areas and potential for risks before an event can occur instead of needing to react to an event in hindsight. Additionally, risk managers need to instill a culture of "if you see something, say something." Staff needs to be encouraged to report observed risks. Creating an environment in which all staff take ownership in the safety and well-being of the facility will help prevent near misses and critical events.

## INFECTION CONTROL AND UNIVERSAL PRECAUTION PROCEDURES

**Infection control** prevents or hinders the spread of infections in healthcare settings. Infections happen when germs get into the body, multiply, and cause an unwanted reaction. Infections require a source. This can be a patient, healthcare worker, or a family member. Germs and infections can come from surfaces such as bed rails, medical equipment, countertops, faucets, and sinks and medical devices such as needles, catheters, and intravenous lines. The germs are then transmitted through contact, fluid sprays and splashes, inhalation, and sharps injuries. **Universal precautions** are in place to attempt to reduce the risk of transmission of bloodborne and other pathogens. Standard precautions include hand hygiene as the most effective way to prevent transmission, including washing and using antimicrobial gel. Additionally, the use of personal protective equipment (gloves, gowns, booties, masks, and eye protection) are the first line of defense for a medical professional.

## MONITORING SENTINEL EVENTS

A **sentinel event** is an unexpected event that causes physical or psychological injury or death of the party involved. The Joint Commission (JCAHO) calls for every facility to have a policy in place for an immediate investigation. Facilities will then form a root cause analysis, which evaluates the events leading up to the incident. Once the analysis is complete, this will lead to an action plan to create strategies so that an event of a similar nature does not happen again. Although most sentinel events are issues involving medication errors, postoperative infections, or surgical mistakes, sentinel events that could involve therapy would be due to a fall or a wrong-patient, wrong-site issue. This could include not being aware of precautions (sternal, weight-bearing), having a patient fall and get injured because brake locks were not engaged in a chair or a gait belt was not being used, or simply going into a room to see a patient and not checking a wristband and asking the patient their name and treating the wrong patient.

## BASIC FIRST AID TRAINING IN MEDICAL SETTINGS

Basic first aid and cardiopulmonary resuscitation training is required for employees in all medical settings. Emergencies can happen in a split second, and basic first aid skills can be useful especially if you are in a setting or clinic without nursing care or in the field alone such as in a home health setting. The most basic first aid for dislocation, heat exhaustion, and sprains includes the following:

- **Dislocation**: Immediately call 911, and do not move the joint. If you try to force the bones back into place, you may cause permanent damage to the joint. Put ice on the area to help reduce swelling.
- **Heat exhaustion**: Have the person lay down with their feet up out of the heat and in a shady or air-conditioned area. Have them drink cool water or something with electrolytes (Gatorade, Pedialyte) while applying cool compresses and fanning. Monitor for agitation, confusion, vomiting, and inability to drink.
- **Sprain**: Follow the rest, ice, compression, elevation (RICE) protocol: Have the person sit and rest the injured area, ice the area immediately for 15 to 20 minutes, compress the area with an elastic or ACE bandage, and elevate the injured above the heart.
- **Anaphylaxis:** A life-threatening allergic reaction to allergy-causing substance (peanuts, bee stings, shell fish). Immediately call 911, administer the epinephrine autoinjector, and write the time of injection on the person's arm in pen for the paramedics. Have the person lie still on his back.
- **Burn**: A burn is tissue damage from chemicals, sun, radiation, or contact with fire. Immediately call 911 if it is a deep or large wound. For a significant burn, remove the burned person from danger while keeping yourself safe (make sure that the power source is off in an electrical burn), make sure the person is breathing, remove any restrictive or smoldering clothing, cover the burn with a moist bandage, and elevate the area while monitoring for shock. For a minor burn, hold the burned area under cool water and remove any restrictive clothing and jewelry. DO NOT break any blisters, and bandage the wound with a clean, dry bandage.
- **Cut**: Make sure that your hands are clean. Apply pressure to stop the bleeding. Clean and rinse the wound with water. Apply an antibiotic gel that is in your first aid kit, and cover the wound with a bandage.

## PRECAUTIONS FOR EARLY MOBILIZATION IN THE CRITICALLY ILL AND ICU PATIENTS

Early mobilization in the intensive care unit (ICU) is currently an emerging area of research. This is a change in the culture for the ICU, which used to be one of letting a patient rest in bed and keeping them as relaxed and immobile as possible to facilitate healing and medical stability. The benefits of early mobilization include reduced hospital acquired weakness, improved functional recovery within the hospital, improved mobility at facility discharge, and reduced hospital length of stay. Early mobilization requires a multidisciplinary team approach with frequent concurrent treatments with PT/OT and respiratory in addition to nursing staff. Precautions will mainly be based on labs being stable as well as stability with respiratory issues. Additionally, having enough people present to assist the patient and to manage lines including the ventilator is key. Most ICU treatment will be bed-based, edge-of-bed, or simple transfers to a chair at the bedside. Edge-of-bed activity can be any of the following:

- trunk control activity (leaning and reaching outside of the base of support and returning to the midline)
- seated ADLs (tooth brushing, face washing, combing hair, cleaning glasses)
- vestibular training (change of gaze, weight shifting)
- joint compression
- ROM
- lung expansion/deep-breathing activity
- cognitive activity
- endurance.

## PRECAUTIONS AND CONTRAINDICATIONS AFTER CARDIAC SURGERY

Heart disease is the leading cause of death in the United States. The most common way to treat coronary heart disease is with open heart surgery, in which the sternum is cut and the chest is split open for access to the heart. Sternal precautions are used after open heart surgery to avoid pulling apart and opening the sternum incision as it is healing. Patients are advised to keep a small pillow nearby to hug for counter pressure if they need to cough or sneeze. Patients are taught how to log roll while hugging a pillow to transition from lying to sitting, only pushing up with the elbows, and they are shown techniques to stand using only the legs to push up and using the arms for balance only. Sternal precautions are advised for the first 6–8 weeks after surgery. Sternal precautions include the following:

- **Do not lift more than 5–8 lb** (a gallon of milk is 8 lbs). This means no housework, hunting, meal prep, lifting pots and pans, carrying groceries or laundry, or lifting children or pets.
- **No pushing or pulling with your arms**. Opening a French door refrigerator requires modification, getting out of bed, opening a heavy door, pushing a grocery cart, cannot propel a wheelchair.
- **Do not reach behind your back or reach both arms out to the side**. Modifications are needed for peri care, dressing, and reaching for things on a bedside table.
- **Do not reach both arms overhead**. Kitchen plates and dishes need to be easily accessible on a counter; things on high shelves need to be moved down lower.

## PRECAUTIONS AND CONTRAINDICATIONS BASED ON THE LAB WORK OF PATIENTS

Critical thinking and clinical decision making are key components to being a licensed healthcare professional. When working in an acute care setting, lab values become a key part of an intervention to determine the safety of a therapy treatment. A bad lab value can determine if you will see a patient, or whether you're going to hold therapy. It is important to not only look at the actual lab number, but to notice trends over the last few blood draws. The following are the most critical labs that need to be checked prior to the start of treatment:

|  | Female | Male | No exercise | Light exercise | Resistive exercise |
|---|---|---|---|---|---|
| HCT | 37%–48% | 39%–55% | <25% | 25%–30% | >30% |
| HGB (g/mL) | 12.2–14.7 | 13.9–18.0 | <8 | 8–10 | >10 |
| WBC per mm³ | 4,500–11,000 | 4,500–11,000 | <5,000 with fever | >5,000 | >5,000 as tolerated |

123

| | Female | Male | No exercise | Light exercise | Resistive exercise |
|---|---|---|---|---|---|
| **Platelets per uL** | 150,000–400,000 | 150,000–400,000 | <20,000 | 20,000–50,000 | >50,000 |
| **Troponin U/L** | <0.04 | <0.04 | >0.02 | 0.05–0.2; check trends | N/A |

## PRECAUTIONS AND CONTRAINDICATIONS AFTER SPINAL SURGERY

The most common types of back surgeries are laminectomy, discectomy, fusion, kyphoplasty, and vertebroplasty. The following is a list of precautions and contraindications for each type of procedure. Patients recovering from back surgery are given "BLT precautions" and are educated that they are not allowed to bend, lift, or twist. Lifting more than 8 lb is discouraged (a gallon of milk weighs 8 lb). These patients will have some type of back brace protocol and will usually be required to wear a brace at all times. Patients are advised to change positions often and are encouraged to walk frequently. Patients are taught log roll techniques for getting out of bed; instructed to not cross their knees or ankles while sitting, standing, or lying down; and to place a pillow between the knees while sleeping for comfort and to keep the spine in good alignment.

### COMMON SPINAL SURGERIES

The following are common spinal surgeries:

- *Kyphoplasty*: Performed after a compression fracture in order to stabilize the fracture and to restore the height that was lost by the vertebral fracture. A balloon is inserted into the fractured bone to create space, and then it is filled with cement.
- *Vertebroplasty*: Performed after a compression fracture in order to stabilize the fracture and to restore the height that was lost by the vertebral fracture. The difference between the vertebroplasty and kyphoplasty is that instead of a balloon being used to create space for the cement, the cement is placed into the fracture of the bone.
- *Laminectomy*: Also called decompression surgery. Removes lamina to enlarge the spinal canal to relieve pressure on the spinal cord or nerves.
- *Discectomy*: Removes the damaged portion of a herniated disk to avoid cord and nerve compression.
- *Spinal fusion*: This procedure fuses two joints together into one structure in the back. This is common after a fracture, degenerative disk disease, or stenosis.

## TREATING AN OBSERVATION PATIENT AND THE TWO-MIDNIGHT RULE

When a patient is admitted into a hospital, they are given a status. It can be inpatient or observation. As inpatient status means that the patient is formally admitted to the hospital with a doctor's order. If a patient is under **observation status**, they are considered outpatient status, which means that the physician is keeping them under close supervision to determine if they are sick enough to need inpatient treatment. Even though they are staying overnight in the facility and receiving treatment from staff, things are coded differently and it is not considered an inpatient admission. This becomes problematic should a patient need to discharge to an SNF. Medicare and most insurance will not pay for SNF placement with a hospitalization on observation status. The patient must be inpatient status. The **two-midnight rule** states that inpatient hospital admission under Medicare that lasts less than two midnights must be treated and billed as outpatient, or observation status. Any "midnight" on observation status does not count toward the three-day qualifying hospital stay for SNF placement.

## 8-MINUTE MEDICARE RULE

The **8-minute rule** is for timed-based CPT codes. It states that in order to receive payment from Medicare, a therapist needs to provide intervention for at least 8 minutes. This does not apply to the untimed codes used for evaluations, reevaluations, or untimed modalities. This applies only to timed modalities such as therapeutic exercises, therapeutic activity, ADLs, etc. During each session, Medicare looks at the total minutes of skilled, one-on-one therapy provided by the practitioner and divides that total minutes by 15. If 8 or more minutes are left over, you can bill for one more additional unit. If seven or fewer minutes remain, you cannot bill an additional unit and the time is considered lost.

**Time = Units**
0– 7 minutes = 0 units
8– 22 minutes = 1 unit
23– 37 minutes = 2 units
38– 52 minutes = 3 units
53– 67 minutes = 4 units
68– 82 minutes = 5 units

## MDS

The **Minimum Data Set (MDS)** is a process for assessment of all residents in Medicare- or Medicaid-certified nursing homes. The MDS categorizes a patient's functional abilities, and it is a significant part of the way that Medicare and Medicaid provide reimbursement and monitor the quality of care provided to SNF residents. Staff must complete the MDS for each resident within 14 days of admission and again each year. The MDS must be reviewed every 3 months, and it must be reassessed whenever there is a major change in the patient's condition.

## NPI

A **National Provider Identifier (NPI)** number is 10-digit identification number issued to healthcare providers and organizations by the federal government for identification and billing purposes across payment sources. NPIs are issued by the National Plan and Provider Enumeration System. If you are a Health Insurance Portability and Accountability Act of 1996-covered practitioner or if you are a healthcare provider/supplier who bills Medicare for your services, you need an NPI number. NPI numbers do not expire nor do they need to be updated. The number will be deactivated if the practitioner dies or closes their practice. NPI numbers are further classified by a taxonomy code. Healthcare Provider Taxonomy Codes are descriptors that categorizes the type, classification, and specialty of the healthcare providers. The taxonomy code for occupational therapy is 225X00000X. This code can be further organized by code categories to designate the area of practice: pediatric, gerontology, mental health, etc.

## THERAPY REIMBURSEMENT STRUCTURES

There are three forms of reimbursement in healthcare: fee for service (FFS), capitation, and bundled/episode-based payments. An FFS reimbursement is a payment that is based on what procedures the practitioner provides. Each individual item that a patient receives is coded with a price attached, and the payment is made based on an à la carte price. Capitation is a payment that will cover all services for a medical episode over a specific period of time. If the provider has a deal with an insurance company for $100 a month, the beneficiary can be seen as many times as they want and receive as many services as they need, but the provider will still only receive $100 a month. Bundled/Episode-based payment is reimbursement based on the expected costs for defined episodes of care. If the expected cost of an orthopedic procedure is $10,000, all of the patient's care including hospital stay, surgery, therapy, etc. needs to stay within or less than the $10,000 because that is all the reimbursement that will be provided. If the facility spends more, they will lose money on that case.

## MEDICARE VS. MEDICAID

**Medicare** is a federally funded program that provides health coverage despite income if you are 65 and older or have a documented and severe disability. **Medicaid** is a federal-state program that varies state to state that provides health coverage to anyone that has a significantly low income. You can apply for Medicaid is you have mounting medical expenses that you cannot afford or if you are you are pregnant, under age 18 or over age 65, blind, or disabled. Not all nursing homes, assisted living facilities, or clinics will accept Medicaid payments, or they may have a cap on the number of patients with Medicaid that they will take at any given time because the reimbursement rate is lower than most other payers.

## THERAPY REIMBURSEMENT TERMS

Therapy services are impacted dramatically by documenting, billing, and payer regulations. The ability for a facility to get reimbursed for therapy treatment is paramount to the success and stability of a therapy program. The following terms are important definitions in the billing process:

| Term | Definition |
| --- | --- |
| **Medical necessity** | Treatment, services, or supplies needed to prevent, diagnose, or treat an illness, injury, or condition and the symptoms related to it. |
| **Beneficiary** | The person eligible for the benefits in a healthcare program or insurance policy. |
| **Benefit period** | The length of time during which a benefit is paid. It begins the day that you are admitted to a hospital or skilled nursing facility (SNF) and ends when you have not received care in an inpatient hospital or skilled care in an SNF for 60 consecutive days. |
| **Dual eligibility** | A person qualifies for Medicare and Medicaid benefits simultaneously. |
| **Spend down** | In order to qualify for Medicaid, some people need to spend down their excess and surplus income on medical bills before medical benefits can be approved. Medicaid rules vary from state to state. In general, a single/widowed individual can retain $2,000 in assets, and married couples who are still living together can retain $3,000 in assets. |
| **Fee for service** | A payment model in which services are paid for individually or à la carte and not bundled together. |
| **Capitation** | A payment model in which a provider of facility is paid a fixed amount per patient for a prescribed period of time by an insurer. |
| **Cost-based reimbursement** | A payment model in which the insurance company will make payments to providers and facilities based on the costs of the care provided to the beneficiary. |
| **Third-party payer** | A payment model in which an organization pays medical claims on behalf of the insured beneficiary. |

## ICD-10 CODES

**International Classification of Diseases (ICD-10)** codes is a system used by healthcare providers to classify and code all diagnoses, symptoms, and procedures of a patient as part of the billing process. The codes provide detailed information and greater specificity for the reasons that a therapist is seeing a patient. The codes support medical necessity in documentation, which can affect whether or not the payer will reimburse the claim. The medical diagnosis codes are assigned by a physician, and a therapist or rehabilitation manager will often choose the treating diagnosis code. Therapists need to identify the code for the functional/treating diagnosis to designate the specific deficit that the patient is being seen for. Common ICD-10 codes that are used for occupational therapy are as follows:

- Z91.81 History of falls
- M62.81 Generalized muscle weakness
- R53.1 Weakness
- R53.81 Other malaise/Chronic debility/Debility/General physical deterioration
- R27.9 Unspecified lack of coordination
- R29.3 Abnormal posture.

## G-CODES

The Centers for Medicare & Medicaid Services (CMS) uses **G-codes** to collect information about its beneficiaries' functional limitations. This system was established in 2013 to collect information over the course of therapy services to understand and identify conditions, outcomes, and expenditures. There are 42 functional G-codes. Six of the G-code sets are used by PT and OT, and eight of the G-code sets are for SLP functional limitations. G-codes are documented at evaluation noting current status and goal status. They are required for all Medicare patients at the initial evaluation, on or before the 10th visit/progress note, and again at discharge. Once a G-code is determined, a severity modifier for the function is chosen.

| Code Range | Descriptor |
|---|---|
| G8978-G8980 | Mobility: walking and moving around |
| G8981-G8983 | Changing and maintaining body position |
| G8984-G8986 | Carrying, moving, and handling objects |
| G8987-G8989 | Self-care |
| G8990-G8992 | Other PT/OT primary limitation |
| G8993-G8995 | Other PT/OT subsequent limitation |

The following are the G-codes modifiers used for PT/OT:

| Modifier | Restriction |
|---|---|
| CH | 0% impaired, limited, or restricted |
| CI | At least 1% but less than 20% impaired, limited, or restricted |
| CJ | At least 20% but less than 40% impaired, limited, or restricted |
| CK | At least 40% but less than 60% impaired, limited, or restricted |
| CL | At least 60% but less than 80% impaired, limited, or restricted |
| CM | At least 80% but less than 100% impaired, limited, or restricted |
| CN | 100% impaired, limited, or restricted |

## CPT CODES

The **Current Procedural Terminology (CPT)** is a medical code set that is used to report medical, surgical, and diagnostic procedures in addition to the *ICD-10* codes as part of the billing and reimbursement process. With the exception of evaluations and reevaluations, which are nontimed codes, all other CPT codes are billed in 15-minute intervals based on the Medicare 8-minute rule. The therapist is responsible for identifying what codes they are using to bill that best describe the treatment they provided to their patient. The following are the most common CPT codes used in occupational therapy:

| CPT Code | Descriptor |
|---|---|
| 97165 | Occupational therapy evaluation, low complexity |
| 97166 | Occupational therapy evaluation, moderate complexity |
| 97167 | Occupational therapy evaluation, high complexity |
| 97168 | Reevaluation |
| 97110 | Therapeutic exercise |
| 97112 | Neuromuscular reeducation |
| 97530 | Therapeutic activity |
| 97535 | Self-care/Home management/ADLs |
| 97140 | Manual therapy |

## PAYMENT AND COVERAGE FOR OCCUPATIONAL THERAPY SERVICES

### SERVICES BY MEDICARE

In 2018, Congress eliminated therapy caps. Therapy caps were limits on how much **Medicare** would pay for therapy services in a single calendar year. Medicare Parts A and B both cover occupational therapy services. Medicare Part A is also known as hospital insurance. It helps cover inpatient medical care, including hospitals, SNFs, and occasionally home healthcare. Medicare Part B helps cover medically necessary and preventive outpatient services. Medicare Part C is also known as Medicare Advantage (MA). It covers about one-third of all Medicare beneficiaries. MA plans are sold to private insurance companies that offer Medicare benefits, and they must provide occupational therapy services that are equal to or better than what is offered with Medicare Parts A and B. As a therapist, be diligent about checking with the payer source because each MA plan can charge a patient different copays and deductibles and have different requirements for therapy authorization prior to service.

### SERVICES BY MEDICAID

**Medicaid** is a healthcare program for low-income people that is funded by the states and the federal government. Medicaid is run by the Centers for Medicare & Medicaid Services (CMS), but each state will control how the specific program is run using federal laws as a guide. Occupational therapy along with physical and speech therapy are not mandatory coverages but instead are considered "optional" benefits under Medicaid, allowing each state to choose if they want to cover therapy services.

### SERVICES BY THE VETERANS HEALTH ADMINISTRATION

The **Veterans Health Administration (VHA)** is the largest healthcare system in the country. Any veteran is eligible for care from any VHA doctor or facility, but not all benefits are available to all veterans. Veterans with health insurance can use their private health insurance to supplement their VHA benefits. Many veterans get their insurance through TRICARE. TRICARE is for the healthcare needs of active-duty service members and for retired active-duty service members as well as people retired from the National Guard who are age 60 or older. TRICARE covers services and supplies furnished by authorized providers under the Civilian Health and Medical Program of the Uniformed Services (CHAMPUS). Occupational therapy services are covered by TRICARE only if they are provided by an OT. Services will not be covered or reimbursed if they are provided by an occupational therapy assistant (OTA) because CHAMPUS does not consider OTAs as authorized providers.

## SERVICES BY COMMERCIAL INSURANCE

Many insurance plans cover occupational therapy, but every plan is different. Most cover occupational therapy in an acute care hospital setting, but they may have exclusions in other areas, such as outpatient and school-based therapies. Many insurance plans will allow for short-term occupational therapy if it meets certain criteria or diagnosis standards and is deemed medically necessary. In some cases, the benefits are defined by the total number of sessions covered per year, and some companies will have the beneficiary pay higher deductibles in order to include therapy services.

## THERAPY PAYMENT DENIALS AND THE APPEAL PROCESS

It is not uncommon for therapy treatment to be denied by a provider. The most common reasons for denial are the following:

- Error: Misspelled name, the time is not documented, wrong procedure code, transposing social security or birthday numbers.
- Lack of progress: If the notes are not detailed showing patient progress, claims can be denied.
- Medical necessity: If a case is not made to show explicitly why therapy is indicated, services can be denied.
- Credentialing or provider issues.
- Submission outside a specified time frame.
- Needs a modifier: If PT and OT are providing two completely separate and distinct services during the same treatment period but both are billing the same code (therapeutic exercise, therapeutic activity), a modifier is needed. If the biller does not use a modifier, the claim will likely be denied.

If a claim is denied, most facilities have a billing department that uses a form letter to appeal the process. The biller is responsible for identifying why the claim was denied and then must contact the payer to determine if that is actually why the claim is denied. Then they must follow the detailed instructions for correcting, rebilling, and resubmitting the claim that they are provided. This may include having a therapist make addendums to the notes in order to correct an error.

## ROLE OF AOTA

The **American Occupational Therapy Association (AOTA)** is a national organization for occupational therapy practitioners that was established in 1917. The goal is to represent the interests and concerns of occupational therapy students and practitioners as well as improve and influence the practice of the profession. As an OT, membership is not mandatory; however, AOTA provides networking, discounted continuing education, conference opportunities, professional support, special interest information, discounts on supplies and education, as well as advocacy and information about the field. Students in occupational therapy school are encouraged to join, and there are special forums and meetings during the conference in April just for students and new graduates. Each year in April for National Occupational Therapy Month, a conference is held in a different state. These conferences are a way to complete all the required continuing education for the year in one event as well as provide a place to network, job search, stay abreast of new and emerging practices, and research and present research or therapy techniques.

## ROLE OF ACOTE

The American Occupational Therapy Association's Accreditation Council for Occupational Therapy Education (ACOTE) is an organization that is the accrediting agency for occupational therapy education in the United States. It monitors more than 400 schools for OT and OTA programs in the

United States. It is recognized by the Department of Education and the Council for Higher Education Accreditation. It is the job of ACOTE to designate the minimum standards that schools will have and to ensure the development of quality programs It is ACOTE that has recently mandated that the entry-level degree requirement for the OT will move to the doctoral level by July 2027.

## ROLE OF AOTPAC

A **political action committee (PAC)** is an organization whose goal is raising and spending money to help in electing candidates who meet the interests or needs of a certain organization or cause. The **American Occupational Therapy Political Action Committee (AOTPAC)** is a nonprofit organization made up of members of AOTA that furthers the legislative issues that concern the practice of and practitioners of occupational therapy. They work to support candidates that will further the cause and promote occupational therapy and advocate for political action influencing issues that affect the profession and the healthcare system. Fundraising efforts are also made for candidates running in the U. S. House of Representatives and the U. S. Senate. Participation in AOTPAC is voluntary. The AOTA board of directors appoints six AOTPAC board members to represent the different regions of the United States.

## JCAHO

The **Joint Commission (JCAHO)** is a not-for-profit organization that seeks to improve the quality and standards of healthcare facilities. It is essentially a standard-setting and accrediting organization in healthcare. JCAHO accredits hospitals, doctors' offices, nursing homes, office-based surgery centers, behavioral health treatment facilities, and home health services. Accreditation is 2 years for laboratory settings and 3 years for all other settings. JCAHO accreditation surveys are unannounced. JCAHO surveyors are medical experts in various fields including physicians, nurses, administrators, and allied health professionals. Surveyors select patients randomly and use their medical records as a roadmap to evaluate standards compliance. Surveyors will pick a "tracer." A tracer is a patient they randomly choose to track the patient's experience in the facility. They will talk to the doctors, nurses, and any staff who interacted with the patient. Surveyors will also observe doctors and medical staff providing care. Once a survey is completed, JCAHO has 2 weeks to 2 months to provide results and accreditation.

## CARF

The **Commission on Accreditation of Rehabilitation Facilities (CARF)** is the alternative organization to JCAHO for accreditation. CARF is a nonprofit organization that provides accreditation on a global scale. They accredit aging services, behavioral health clinics, vision rehabilitation centers, employment and community services locations, medical rehabilitation facilities, opioid treatment programs, and career centers. A survey can last up to 3 days to determine how the facility is meeting as many as 1,500 standards set by CARF. They have three levels of accreditation:

- Three-year accreditation: The provider is meeting or exceeding CARF standards.
- One-year accreditation: There are some deficiencies, although the program shows capability and commitment in correcting the issues.
- Provisional accreditation: The provider is still working at the 1-year level longer than 1 year and has not yet met CARF standards. It may face nonaccreditation status.
- Hospitals and facilities need accreditation because it is required in order to get paid from federally funded Medicare and Medicaid programs.

## RUGs

**Resource utilization groups (RUGs)** are a classification system used to determine reimbursement levels for patients in SNFs. In an SNF, data from the MDS are used to determine the RUG category. A resident is assigned to one of the major categories of RUGs based on their functional abilities. The categories are as follows: rehabilitation plus extensive services, rehabilitation, extensive services, special care, special care low, clinically complex, behavioral symptoms and cognitive performance, and reduced physical function. There are then filtered into a five-category RUG-IV payment system:

- Ultra (U) is 720+ minutes of total therapy (PT/OT/SLP):
  - two or more therapies are provided, with 5 days or more per week of one type of therapy and 3 days or more for the second therapy.
- Very high (V) is 500–719 minutes of total therapy (PT/OT/SLP):
  - 5 days or more per week of one type of therapy.
- High (H) is 325–499 minutes of total therapy (PT/OT/SLP):
  - 5 days or more per week of one type of therapy.
- Medium (M) is 150–324 minutes of total therapy (PT/OT/SLP):
  - at least 5 days per week of therapy of any combination.
- Low (L) is 45–149 minutes of total therapy (PT/OT/SLP):
  - at least 3 days per week of therapy of any combination and at least two nursing restorative programs, each administered for at least 15 minutes, each for 6 or more days.

## ROLE DELINEATION BETWEEN AN OTR AND OTA

OTRs spend 3–4 years completing a master's-level education program. They are responsible for the evaluation of patients, setting the treatment plan of care, setting goals, writing progress notes, and completing the discharge. Occupational therapy assistants (OTAs) spend 2 years completing an associate's degree. They are responsible for following the POC established by the OTR and implementing the treatment plan. They are not allowed to complete evaluations or discharges, and their documentation needs to be cosigned. Supervision will vary on a state-to-state basis and will also be based on the comfort level of the OTR because the OTA is practicing under their license.

## REQUIREMENTS FOR SUPERVISION OF A STUDENT OR TECHNICIAN

Supervision of a student will vary based on the setting and comfort level of the OTR; however, there are guidelines specifically set by Medicare to dictate supervision guidelines. The OTR will determine the appropriate manner of supervision of therapy students consistent with state and local laws. For patients that have Medicare Part A and are in a hospital, SNF, or inpatient rehabilitation setting, the OTR will determine the appropriate manner of supervision while maintaining state and local laws. Patients that are on Medicare Part B must be treated by a student within the line of sight of the OTR, and the OTR must remain in the same room. An occupational therapy aide/technician is a support personnel that is unlicensed and assists under the supervision of a licensed OT. Supervision laws will vary on a state-to-state basis and will also be based on the comfort level of the OTR whose license the tech is working under. In most cases, techs are allowed to provide services in the same room as the OTR and are also allowed to go and get a patient and bring him or her to the therapist for treatment.

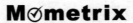

## CLINICAL FIELDWORK EDUCATOR

Becoming a clinical fieldwork educator is an important and meaningful role. The opportunity to help mentor and educate new clinicians coming into the field is an important part of the process of growing the field and shaping the future of occupational therapy. Occupational therapy students are required to complete Levels I and II fieldwork placements. Level I students may be supervised by a licensed OT. A Level II fieldwork student must be supervised by a licensed OT who has been in practice for at least 1 year. There is not a minimum time frame for Level I fieldwork; however, Level II is required to be a minimum of a minimum of 24 weeks with a full-time schedule. Level I fieldwork lets the student develop a basic comfort level with patient care and the therapy process. It is mostly directed observation and participation in selected intervention at the discretion of the OTR. During Level II fieldwork, the student will take on a full caseload with supervision from the OTR and provide learning opportunities and in-service trainings to the staff at the facility. Completion and passing of fieldwork assignments is required in order to sit for the NBCOT exam.

# Sample Scenarios for OT Patients

**YOU ARE EVALUATING A PATIENT WHO HAS A COMPLETE SPINAL CORD INJURY AT THE LEVEL OF C4. BRIEFLY DESCRIBE HIS EXPECTED FUNCTIONAL OUTCOMES, AND THE OT TREATMENT FOCUS.**

A typical C4 tetraplegic will eventually be able to breathe without a vent, though will require some assistance for deep coughing due to lack of innervation of the abdominals and an inability to forcefully exhale. He will be able to elevate his shoulders and will have complete movement of his head. This patient will be dependent in a majority of his self-care tasks and will require a lift for transfers. OT focus for this patient will be to train him in the use of a mouth stick for leisure activities such as reading or using the computer. A straw can also be used for this purpose. He will be able to drink from a container that is set up with a straw in reach. This patient will be able to independently operate a wheelchair with an alternative method of steering, such as sip and puff or head controls. Caregiver education is the primary OT focus, however he should also be taught to self-instruct caregivers on his ADL and transfer routine.

**YOU ARE TREATING A PATIENT WITH A TRAUMATIC BRAIN INJURY, WHO YOU SUSPECT HAS LEFT NEGLECT. DESCRIBE HOW YOU WOULD TEST FOR THIS CONDITION, AND LIST STRATEGIES FOR TREATMENT.**

Initial observation of a patient during ADLS can help determine if neglect is present. If the patient leaves food on only one half of his plate, or does not attempt to dress one side of his body, then neglect is likely. Typical evaluations for neglect involve having the patient bisect a line or draw a clock, both of which will be skewed to the attended side.

A patient with neglect must be taught to regularly attend the affected side, and OT treatment should involve participation in activities that encourage crossing the midline. Caregivers should be educated to approach the patient from the affected side to promote environmental scanning. The OT might even arrange the patient's room so that items regularly sought out will be on his affected side. Cues should be provided regularly until the patient is able to compensate appropriately for the visual deficit.

**DESCRIBE TYPICAL DEFICITS AND OT TREATMENT FOR A PATIENT WITH SEVERE BURNS IN BOTH ARMS.**

A patient with burns is susceptible to decreased ROM due to a rapid rate of collagen formation in the affected area. OTs must perform daily stretching and passive range of motion to decrease the risk for scar band formation. The skin should be moistened with cream, typically cocoa butter, prior to treatment. The stretching should be slow and passive to the point of blanching, or becoming very light in color. Care should be taken not to tear fragile skin, which can increase the risk of infection. The OT may also choose to provide a splint for day or nighttime wear in order to encourage a functional position during healing. The patient should be involved in as many ADL activities as possible to encourage active movement, and caregivers should be educated to follow through with splinting and ROM programs.

**A PATIENT ENTERS YOUR CLINIC WITH SEVERE EDEMA IN HER HAND. REVIEW SOME OF THE POSSIBLE TREATMENTS FOR HER CONDITION, IN ADDITION TO TREATMENTS THAT ARE CONTRAINDICATED.**

Appropriate treatments for a patient with edema are as follows:

Contrast baths, which consist of alternately placing the hand in an ice bath and warm water at intervals of a 1:2 ratio, may be combined with active ROM while the hand is submerged.

Compression garments, string wrapping and ace wraps can encourage fluid to move proximally. Care should be taken to ensure the garments or wrappings are not too tight.

Retrograde massage also encourages fluid re-absorption, and involves slow gentle pressure on the affected extremity, applied distally to proximally. Lymph edema massage is a specialized form of fluid mobilization, however performance of this technique requires specialized training.

Finally, active movement combined with limb elevation is an appropriate treatment that can be carried out by the patient and her caregiver outside of the clinic.

Activities which should be avoided when treating edema are direct application of heat, which can encourage further fluid collection due to vasodilatation, and aggressive ROM exercises which can further aggravate inflammatory response.

### DESCRIBE THE OT COURSE OF TREATMENT FOR A PATIENT WHO HAS RECENTLY HAD A BELOW THE ELBOW AMPUTATION IN HIS DOMINANT ARM. HE IS EXPERIENCING HYPERSENSITIVITY IN THE AFFECTED LIMB, AND HAS A GOAL OF USING A PROSTHETIC LIMB FOR FUNCTIONAL TASKS.

Hypersensitivity and phantom pain are common in the distal stump of recently amputated limbs. In order to prepare this patient for the eventual use of a prosthetic, the stump must be subjected to desensitization. This involves increasing the sensory tolerance at the stump site by progressively introducing textures and increasing amounts of pressure. Examples of this are brushing the site with a towel, or pressing the stump into a cushioned surface. As tolerance increases, the OT should introduce rougher textures and firmer surfaces. Preparation for use of an upper extremity prosthetic should also involve active and passive ROM for maximum joint mobility, and strengthening of the muscles that flex and extend the distal joint. Gross coordination training of the proximal joints is also appropriate. The patient can practice using the stump to push objects around a flat surface, or a paintbrush may be strapped to the affected limb.

### YOU ARE SEEING A PATIENT IN THE CLINIC WHO IS UNDERGOING RADIATION FOR BREAST CANCER. SHE PRESENTS WITH DECREASED ROM IN HER UPPER EXTREMITIES AND FATIGUES QUICKLY DURING ADLS. EXPLAIN WHY THESE SYMPTOMS ARE PRESENT, AND OUTLINE THE APPROPRIATE OT INTERVENTION.

In patients undergoing breast cancer treatment, it is common for radiation to have affected the mobility in the joints near the radiation site. Soft tissues in the surrounding areas are often at risk for "radiation fibrosis" which can last for years, even after treatment is complete. Patients with symptoms of decreased ROM and a feeling of stiffness will benefit from mobilization of the affected joints and passive ROM. Heat and ultrasound are contraindicated in patients with cancer, as they can accelerate spread of the tumor cells. Decreased endurance is also common in patients undergoing cancer treatment, and should be addressed through education about energy conservation and work simplification techniques. Providing adaptive equipment to ease the performance of ADLs can assist with these techniques. Examples of appropriate adaptive equipment include but are not limited to a shower chair, a reacher, or bedside commode.

**DURING THE INITIAL EVALUATION, YOUR PATIENT WITH A COMPLETE C6 TETRAPLEGIA HAS ESTABLISHED A GOAL OF BEING ABLE TO FEED HERSELF INDEPENDENTLY, WITH THE LEAST AMOUNT OF EQUIPMENT POSSIBLE. CURRENTLY, SHE HAS 3/5 STRENGTH FOR SHOULDER FLEXION, AND 3+/5 FOR ELBOW FLEXION. FINGER FLEXION IS ABSENT. DESCRIBE THE STAGES OF PROGRESSING THIS PATIENT TO HER GOAL.**

The initial OT focus should be strength and endurance of shoulder flexion, to ensure hand to mouth movements can be sustained for the duration of the feeding task. If the patient fatigues quickly, she may be initially provided with a mobile arm support to assist in feeding. In the absence if finger flexion, a universal cuff can allow her to hold a utensil, using a plate guard as a barrier for spill-free scooping. A cup with a large handle or a long straw can be provided to ease drinking. As shoulder strength progresses, the mobile arm support should be discontinued. The OT should also focus on increasing the strength of tenodesis grasp in order to allow the patient to hold a utensil without a cuff. A built-up handle for the utensil may be necessary initially or permanently. In order to make eating more efficient, the OT should focus on strengthening the specific movements that ease scooping or stabbing food, bringing the hand to the mouth and releasing the hand after biting.

**DESCRIBE THE DIFFERENCES BETWEEN THE TYPICAL BEHAVIORS OF A PATIENT WHO IS AT AN ALLEN COGNITIVE LEVEL OF 2.4-2.8 VERSUS A PATIENT WHO IS 3.8-4.0.**

In Allen level 2.4-2.8, or late dementia, patients still have the gross motors skills required to walk. They tend to wander, or participate in repetitive motions like rocking. In general, they are not able to perform appropriate actions on objects such as articles of clothing. They can respond to simple cues related to movement, such as instruction to stand up after toileting. Usually patients at this level can feed themselves finger foods and self-administer beverages.

At level 3.8-4.0, or early dementia, patients can complete basic self-care skills in a routine. They have deficits in problem solving, and are unable to get past roadblocks in their basic routines. For instance, a patient who runs out of toilet paper might attempt to clean himself with his hand. Patients at this level cannot be reasoned with, and may become agitated if given too much information to process. They are able to learn new skills with repetition.

**YOU ARE TREATING A PATIENT ON A DEMENTIA UNIT WHO IS AT ALLEN COGNITIVE LEVEL 4.4. HER CAREGIVER STATES THAT SHE WAS ABLE TO COMPLETE HER ADLS AT HOME, HOWEVER SHE HAS BEEN DEPENDENT SINCE HER ADMISSION TO THE UNIT. LIST SEVERAL STRATEGIES THAT MIGHT INCREASE THIS PATIENT'S INVOLVEMENT IN HER PERSONAL CARE.**

One of the first things the therapist should do is to find out the patient's former ADL routine from the caregiver, including start time, time needed to complete, and basic setup at home. Next, the therapist should simulate these conditions as closely as possible to maximize the patient's involvement. Some strategies that might encourage greater participation include placing all ADL items in plain view at eye level in the area where they will be used. Clothing choices should be minimized, or pre-arranged outfits should be set out for the patient. Also, extra time should be allowed for this patient to complete her routine. Once an appropriate routine is established, the therapist should ensure that caregivers on the unit are educated regarding the patient's ADL abilities.

**A PATIENT IN HIS THIRTIES IS REFUSING TREATMENT, STATING THAT HIS WIFE WILL DRESS HIM AT HOME. HIS WIFE WORKS FULL-TIME, AND HE DOES NOT QUALIFY FOR HOMECARE ASSISTANCE. THE PATIENT APPEARS TO BE DEPRESSED. DESCRIBE WHAT APPROACH THE OT SHOULD TAKE TO ENCOURAGE PARTICIPATION.**

A patient who appears to be depressed should be referred to a counselor or social worker, and a description of his mood and actions should be passed along to the treating nurses and physicians. In order to encourage the patient to participate, the OT should explain the reasoning behind the treatment she is providing. She should never try to force the patient to do something he does not want to do; however, she should try to find a common ground with him. The next step should be to establish goals with the patient, to determine what is important to him. A patient who is working towards his own personal goal will be more likely to participate that a patient whose established goal does not inspire him. Once the patient is cooperating more, the therapist should set several goals that are quickly achievable. The patient should be reminded of his progress, and mood should be monitored for changes.

### GIVE EXAMPLES OF HOW TO MAKE THE TASK OF PREPARING A SANDWICH SIMPLER OR MORE DEMANDING ON A PATIENT'S PHYSICAL AND COGNITIVE ABILITIES.

To grade thus task so that it will be easier for the client physically, the OT can do any of the following things: place ingredients on a shelf within reach, use adaptive devices such as a built-up knife or jar opener, allow the patient to sit, move items closer to the patient, allow the patient to take breaks, or remove appropriate items from packaging. Cognitively, the OT can reduce the number of ingredient choices, provide instruction during each step, cue for location of items, provide a checklist, or allow extra time for completion of the task

To grade the activity so that it is more difficult physically, the OT might have the patient stand, retrieve the ingredients from various locations, open containers and packaging without assistance, or complete within an allotted time frame. To make it more challenging cognitively, she may ask the patient to complete the task without instruction, or provide multi-step cues and directions. The OT can also ask the patient to locate the ingredients, and to recall safety without cues.

### YOU ARE TREATING A PATIENT WITH MS WHOSE MAIN GOAL IS TO SHOWER IN HER BATHTUB WITH MINIMAL ASSISTANCE. CURRENTLY, SHE CAN TOLERATE 5 MINUTES OF ACTIVITY AT A TIME AND REQUIRES MODERATE ASSISTANCE TO STAND AND TRANSFER. DESCRIBE OT INTERVENTION, INCLUDING USE OF ADAPTIVE DEVICES.

Due to the relapsing and remitting nature of MS, it is important that her therapy and any adaptive equipment provided be appropriate for various levels of the patient's abilities. The first step in OT treatment is to increase her activity tolerance so that a shower will not exhaust her. The patient should participate in endurance training, and dynamic upper body tasks in order to increase tolerance to a more functional level. Next, she should be educated on energy conservation and work simplification. To make showering easier, she can use a tub transfer bench, a long sponge and a handheld shower. The OT should provide training on the use of these items. Caregiver education is also important, as the patient plans to receive some assistance at home. Finally, the OT should complete transfer training and standing tolerance activities to increase the patient's ability with shower transfers, and standing briefly for hygiene.

### YOU ARE EVALUATING A PATIENT WITH AN INCOMPLETE SPINAL CORD INJURY (SCI) AT THE LEVEL C7. DESCRIBE MANUAL MUSCLE AND SENSORY TESTING FOR THIS PATIENT, INCLUDING VARIATIONS TO BE EXPECTED FROM A PATIENT WITH A COMPLETE INJURY AT THE SAME LEVEL.

When completing a sensory or motor test with a patient who has SCI, the patient should be in supine in bed or on a mat, wearing non-restrictive clothing. This will enable the OT to fully access the upper extremities, and to perform both gravity-eliminated and against gravity measurements of muscle strength. The patient's sensation should be measured for deficits in the detection of light touch and pain (a pin prick) in accordance with dermatomes.

A patient with an SCI at C7, who has no other upper extremity injuries, would be expected to have at least fair strength in biceps, triceps, wrist extensors and finger flexors. Sensation should be intact to the C7 dermatome on the lateral forearm. A patient with an incomplete injury may have deficits in sensation and strength at the site of injury, however areas tested below the injury may be partially intact on one or both sides of the body.

**YOU ARE WORKING WITH A CLIENT WHO HAS RIGHT HEMIPARESIS. HE IS ABLE TO STAND WITH SUPERVISION USING A BAR FOR SUPPORT, AND IS INDEPENDENT WITH WHEELCHAIR MOBILITY. HE CAN TOLERATE 20 MINUTES OF ACTIVITY BEFORE NEEDING TO REST. HE LIVES WITH HIS WIFE, WHO CAN PROVIDE LIMITED PHYSICAL ASSISTANCE AT HOME. HIS GOAL IS TO BE AS INDEPENDENT AS POSSIBLE WITH HIS SELF-CARE. DESCRIBE THE ADAPTIVE EQUIPMENT THAT WOULD BE APPROPRIATE FOR THIS PATIENT.**

The patient should go home at a wheelchair level for safety, and thus a lightweight wheelchair should be provided to allow for easy car transport for outings and doctor's appointments. Grooming skills can be performed at the sink from the wheelchair. A suction brush may be appropriate for nail care. The patient may benefit from the use of a reacher during dressing tasks, and to safely access fallen items. A long shoehorn and a dressing stick can decrease the demands of dressing tasks, as can the use of Velcro, elastic shoelaces, and a button hook. A raised toilet seat and a shower chair in conjunction with installation of grab bars are recommended for the bathroom. The patient will also benefit from a handheld shower, as well as long sponge to ease washing of the non-affected extremity. Non-slip surfaces should be used in the shower and on the bathroom floor to decrease the risk of falls.

**YOU ARE TREATING AN ELDERLY PATIENT IN A SUB-ACUTE CARE SETTING WHO HAS SUFFERED A SEVERE CVA. HE HAS REACHED A PLATEAU, AND REQUIRES MODERATE TO MAXIMAL ASSISTANCE WITH HIS ADLs AND TRANSFERS. HIS WIFE SAYS SHE WOULD LIKE TO TAKE HIM HOME. DESCRIBE THE NEXT APPROPRIATE STEPS TO TAKE IN YOUR TREATMENT.**

This patient will require a great deal of physical help at home, and may require even more help when he is fatigued at the end of the day. Maintaining this level of physical activity is taxing on a caregiver, especially an elderly female. The first step for the OT should be to provide direct family training in all aspects of the patient's self-care needs. The spouse should begin to assist with the patient's dressing and bathing, toileting tasks and transfers. The OT's role is to determine whether she is able to safety care for the patient. The next step is to refer the patient to the social worker, who provide advice about community resources to ease the caregiver burden, such as a bath aide. The social worker can also discuss other options for care, and provide any necessary counseling. Often, elderly spouses feel a strong sense of responsibility to care for their loved ones, but it is up to the team to determine whether or not this will meet the patient's needs.

# Special Report: NBCOT Sample Questions

1. An occupational therapist is working in an outpatient orthopedic clinic. During the patient's history the patient reports, "I tore 3 of my 4 Rotator cuff muscles in the past." Which of the following muscles cannot be considered as possibly being torn?

   a. Teres minor
   b. Teres major
   c. Supraspinatus
   d. Infraspinatus

2. An occupational therapist at an outpatient clinic is returning phone calls that have been made to the clinic. Which of the following calls should have the highest priority for medical intervention?

   a. A home health patient reports, "I am starting to have breakdown of my heels."
   b. A patient that received an upper extremity cast yesterday reports, "I can't feel my fingers in my right hand today."
   c. A young female reports, "I think I sprained my ankle about 2 weeks ago."
   d. A middle-aged patient reports, "My knee is still hurting from the TKR."

3. An occupational therapist is assessing a rupture of the ulnar collateral ligament of the thumb. Which of the following terms is another phrase for this condition?

   a. Mallet finger
   b. Gamekeeper's thumb.
   c. Heberden's nodes
   d. Early signs of CTS.

4. An occupational therapist is performing a screening on a patient that has been casted recently on the left upper extremity. Which of the following statements should the occupational therapist be most concerned about?

   a. The patient reports, "I didn't keep my extremity elevated like the doctor asked me to."
   b. The patient reports, "I have been having pain in my left forearm."
   c. The patient reports, "My left arm has really been itching."
   d. The patient reports, "The arthritis in my wrists is flaring up, when I put weight on my crutch."

5. A 93-year-old female with a history of Alzheimer's Disease gets admitted to an Alzheimer's unit. The patient has exhibited signs of increased confusion and limited stability with gait. Moreover, the patient is refusing to use a w/c. Which of the following is the most appropriate course of action for the occupational therapist?

   a. Recommend the patient remain in her room at all times.
   b. Recommend family members bring pictures to the patient's room.
   c. Recommend a speech therapy consult to the doctor.
   d. Recommend the patient attempt to walk pushing the w/c for safety.

6. An occupational therapist is covering a pediatric unit and is responsible for a 15-year-old male patient on the floor. The mother of the child states, "I think my son is sexually interested in girls." The most appropriate course of action of the occupational therapist is to respond by stating:

   a. "I will talk to the doctor about it."
   b. "Has this been going on for a while?"
   c. "How do you know this?"
   d. "Teenagers often exhibit signs of sexual interest in females."

7. An occupational therapist is caring for a patient who has recently been diagnosed with fibromyalgia and COPD. Which of the following tasks should the occupational therapist delegate to an aide?

   a. Transferring the patient during the third visit.
   b. Evaluating the patient
   c. Taking the patient's vital sign while setting up an exercise program
   d. Educating the patient on monitoring fatigue

8. An occupational therapist has been instructed to provide hand wound care for a patient that has active TB and HIV. The occupational therapist should where which of the following safety equipment?

   a. Sterile gloves, mask, and goggles
   b. Surgical cap, gloves, mask, and proper shoewear
   c. Double gloves, gown, and mask
   d. Goggles, mask, gloves, and gown

9. Which of the following correctly identifies the TAM score?

   a. The total of a finger's flexion measurements minus the total extension measurements.
   b. The total of a finger's extension measurements minus the total flexion measurements.
   c. The total of a finger's flexion measurements minus the total extension measurements divided by 2.
   d. The total of a finger's extension measurements minus the total flexion measurements divided by 2.

10. A 64-year-old Alzheimer's patient has exhibited excessive cognitive decline resulting in harmful behaviors. The physician orders restraints to be placed on the patient. Which of the following is the appropriate procedure?

    a. Secure the restraints to the bed rails on all extremities.
    b. Notify the physician that restraints have been placed properly.
    c. Communicate with the patient and family the need for restraints.
    d. Position the head of the bed at a 45-degree angle.

11. A 22-year-old patient in a mental health lock-down unit under suicide watch appears happy about being discharged. Which of the following is probably happening?

    a. The patient is excited about being around family again.
    b. The patient's suicide plan has probably progressed.
    c. The patient's plans for the future have been clarified.
    d. The patient's mood is improving.

12. A patient that has delivered a 8.2 lb. baby boy 3 days ago via c-section, reports white patches on her breast that aren't going away. Which of the following medications may be necessary?

   a. Nystatin
   b. Atropine
   c. Amoxil
   d. Lortab

13. A 64-year-old male who has been diagnosed with COPD, and CHF. The patient exhibits an increase in total body weight of 10 lbs. over the last few days during inpatient therapy. The occupational therapist should:

   a. Contact the patient's physician immediately.
   b. Check the intake and output on the patient's flow sheet.
   c. Encourage the patient to ambulate to reduce lower extremity edema.
   d. Check the patient's vitals every 2 hours.

14. A patient that has TB can be taken off restrictions after which of the following parameters have been met?

   a. Negative culture results.
   b. After 30 days of isolation.
   c. Normal body temperature for 48 hours.
   d. Non-productive cough for 72 hours.

15. An occupational therapist teaching a patient with COPD pulmonary exercises should do which of the following?

   a. Teach purse-lip breathing techniques.
   b. Encourage repetitive heavy lifting exercises that will increase strength.
   c. Limit exercises based on respiratory acidosis.
   d. Take breaks every 10-20 minutes with exercises.

16. A patient asks an occupational therapist the following question. Exposure to TB can be identified best with which of the following procedures?

   a. Chest x-ray
   b. Mantoux test
   c. Breath sounds examination
   d. Sputum culture for gram-negative bacteria

17. A twenty-one-year-old man suffered a concussion during therapy and the MD ordered a MRI. The patient asks, "Will they allow me to sit up during the MRI?" The correct response by the occupational therapist should be.

   a. "I will have to talk to the doctor about letting you sit upright during the test."
   b. "You will be positioned in the reverse Trendelenburg position to maximize the view of the brain."
   c. "The radiologist will let you know."
   d. "You will have to lie down on your back during the test."

18. A fifty-five-year-old man suffered a left frontal lobe CVA. Which of the following should the occupational therapist watch most closely for?

   a. Changes in emotion and behavior
   b. Monitor loss of hearing
   c. Observe appetite and vision deficits
   d. Changes in facial muscle control

19. An occupational therapist working in a pediatric clinic observes bruises on the body of a four-year-old boy. The parents report the boy fell riding his bike. The bruises are located on his posterior chest wall and gluteal region. The occupational therapist should:

   a. Suggest a script for counseling for the family to the doctor on duty.
   b. Recommend a warm bath for the boy to decrease healing time.
   c. Notify the case manager in the clinic about possible child abuse concerns.
   d. Recommend ROM to the patient's spine to decrease healing time.

20. A 14-year-old boy has been admitted to a mental health unit for observation and treatment for a broken wrist and shoulder. The boy becomes agitated and starts yelling at staff members. What should the occupational therapist first response be?

   a. Create an atmosphere of seclusion for the boy according to procedures.
   b. Remove other patients from the area via wheelchairs for added speed.
   c. Ask the patient, "What is making you mad?"
   d. Ask the patient, "Why are you doing this, have you thought about what your parents might say?"

21. An occupational therapist is instructing a patient on the order of sensations with the application of an ice water bath for a swollen L wrist. Which of the following is the correct order of sensations experienced with an ice water bath?

   a. cold, burning, aching, and numbness
   b. burning, aching, cold, and numbness
   c. aching, cold, burning and numbness
   d. cold, aching, burning and numbness

22. An occupational therapist wants to test a patient's ability to sweat. Which of the following assessment tools or techniques would be used?

   a. heated whirlpool
   b. ninhydrin test
   c. tuning fork
   d. counter hydration test

23. An occupational therapist assesses a 43 year carpenter that has recently broken 70% of the bones in his right upper extremity. The carpenter is insistent upon returning to work at the end of the week and being cleared by OT for full duties. Which of the following categories would the patient be placed in on the disability adjustment stage?

   a. Acceptance
   b. Grieving
   c. Anger
   d. Denial

**24. Tricyclics (Antidepressants) sometimes have which of the following adverse effects on patients that have a diagnosis of depression?**

    a.  Shortness of breath
    b.  Fainting
    c.  Large Intestine ulcers
    d.  Distal muscular weakness

**25. An occupational therapist is instructing a patient about the warning signs of (Digitalis) side effects. Which of the following side effects should the occupational therapist tell the patient are sometimes associated with excessive levels of Digitalis?**

    a.  Seizures
    b.  Muscle weakness
    c.  Depression
    d.  Anxiety

**26. An occupational therapist is assessing a patient in an acute care setting. The patient has the following signs: weak pulse, quick respiration, acetone breath, and nausea. Which of the following conditions is most likely occurring?**

    a.  Hypoglycemic patient
    b.  Hyperglycemic patient
    c.  Cardiac arrest
    d.  End-stage renal failure

**27. Medical records indicate a patient has developed a condition of respiratory alkalosis. Which of the following clinical signs would not apply to a condition of respiratory alkalosis?**

    a.  Muscle tetany
    b.  Syncope
    c.  Numbness
    d.  Anxiety

**28. Which of the following lab values would indicate symptomatic AIDS in the medical chart? (T4 cell count per deciliter)**

    a.  Greater than 1000 cells per deciliter
    b.  Less than 500 cells per deciliter
    c.  Greater than 2000 cells per deciliter
    d.  Less than 200 cells per deciliter

**29. An occupational therapist is assessing a patient that has undergone a recent CABG. The occupational therapist notices a mole with irregular edges with a bluish color. The occupational therapist should:**

    a.  Recommend a dermatological consult to the MD.
    b.  Note the location of the mole and contact the physician via the telephone.
    c.  Note the location of the mole and follow-up with the attending physician via the medical record and phone call.
    d.  Remove the mole with a sharp's debridement technique.

30. An occupational therapist is assessing a 18 year-old female who has recently suffered a TBI. The occupational therapist notes a slower pulse and impaired respiration. The occupational therapist should report these findings immediately to the physician, due to the possibility the patient is experiencing which of the following conditions?

    a.  Increased intracranial pressure
    b.  Increased function of cranial nerve X
    c.  Sympathetic response to activity
    d.  Meningitis

31. An occupational therapist is making discharge recommendations to patient that has recently been diagnosed with COPD, Arthritis, and an Anxiety disorder. Which of the following recommendations would be the most helpful for the patient to take their medicine correctly?

    a.  A chart that will have the pills and times broken down in the bathroom.
    b.  A pill container that has different time slots.
    c.  A brightly colored pill container to avoid getting lost.
    d.  Easy access tops on the medication and large labels on the containers.

32. An occupational therapist has been assigned a patient who has recently been diagnosed with Guillain-Barre' Syndrome. Which of the following statements is the most applicable when discussing the impairments with Guillain-Barre' Syndrome with the patient?

    a.  Guillain-Barre' Syndrome gets better after 5 years in almost all cases.
    b.  Guillain-Barre' Syndrome causes limited sensation in the abdominal region.
    c.  Guillain-Barre' Syndrome causes muscle weakness in the legs.
    d.  Guillain-Barre' Syndrome does not affect breathing in severe cases.

33. An occupational therapist is returning phone calls in a pediatric clinic. Which of the following reports most requires the occupational therapist's immediate attention and phone call?

    a.  A 8-year-old boy has been vomiting and appears to have slower movements and has a history of an atrio-ventricular shunt placement.
    b.  A 10-year-old girl feels a dull pain in her abdomen after doing sit-ups in gym class.
    c.  A 7-year-old boy has been having a low fever and headache for the past 3 days that has history of an anterior hand wound.
    d.  A 7-year-old girl that had a cast on her right wrist is complaining of itching.

34. An occupational therapist is assessing a patient in the rehab unit. The patient has suffered a TBI 3 weeks ago. Which of the following is the most distinguishing characteristic of a neurological disturbance?

    a.  LOC (level of consciousness)
    b.  Short term memory
    c.  + Babinski sign
    d.  + Clonus sign

**35. A patient is currently having a petit mal seizure in the clinic on the floor. Which of the following criteria has the highest priority in this situation?**

    a. Provide a safe environment free of obstructions in the immediate area
    b. Call a code
    c. Contact the patient's physician
    d. Prevent excessive movement of the extremities

**36. An occupational therapist is caring for a patient in the step-down unit. The patient has signs of increased intracranial pressure. Which of the following is not a sign of increased intracranial pressure?**

    a. Bradycardia
    b. Increased pupil size bilaterally
    c. Change in LOC
    d. Vomiting

**37. The charge nurse on a cardiac unit tells you a patient is exhibiting signs of right-sided heart failure. Which of the following would not indicate right-sided heart failure?**

    a. Nausea
    b. Anorexia
    c. Rapid weight gain
    d. SOB (shortness of breath)

**38. A 24-year-old man has been admitted to the hospital due to work-related injury. The patient's wife would like to see the patient's chart. The occupational therapist should:**

    a. Provide the chart to the patient's wife following verbal approval by the patient.
    b. Provide the chart to the patient's wife after consulting with the patient's physician.
    c. Get written approval from the patient prior to providing the wife with chart information and call the MD about the patient's request.
    d. Tell the patient' wife, a copy of the patient's medical record is on-file with medical records.

**39. A 49-year-old female is in rehab for a TBI. Which of the following home tasks would take the greatest amount of problem solving and should be practiced in rehab?**

    a. Reading a book for pleasure.
    b. Practice finding small objects like: car keys.
    c. Grooming and self-care ADLs.
    d. Preparing a simple meal.

**40. A patient has just been prescribed Minipress to control hypertension. The occupational therapist should instruct the patient to be observant of the following:**

    a. Dizziness and light headed sensations
    b. Weight gain
    c. Sensory changes in the lower extremities
    d. Fatigue

**41. An occupational therapist is performing an evaluation on patient's wrist. Which of the following diagnostic terms matches the following information: Extension noted at the PIP joint, Flexion of the MCP and DIP joints. Lateral bands have slipped dorsally at the PIP joint?**

    a. Mallet finger
    b. Swan Neck deformity
    c. Boutonniere's deformity
    d. Claw fingers

**42. A 55-year-old female asks an occupational therapist the following, "Which mineral/vitamin is the most important to prevent progression of osteoporosis. The occupational therapist should state:**

    a. Potassium
    b. Magnesium
    c. Calcium
    d. Vitamin B12

**43. A patient has recently been diagnosed with symptomatic bradycardia. Which of the following medications is the most recognized for treatment of symptomatic bradycardia?**

    a. Questran
    b. Digitalis
    c. Nitroglycerin
    d. Atropine

**44. A patient has recently been prescribed Lidocaine Hydrochloride. Which of the following symptoms may occur with over dosage?**

    a. Memory loss and lack of appetite
    b. Confusion and fatigue
    c. Heightened reflexes
    d. Tinnitus and spasticity

**45. Which of the following recommendations would be the most helpful for someone who has right hemiplegia and is going to a driving program offered by occupational therapy?**

    a. Variable digital and voice controls
    b. Alternate brake position
    c. Hand controls with stick on the L
    d. Use of a spinner knob to aid with steering

**46. A patient has suffered a left CVA and has developed severe hemiparesis resulting in a loss of mobility. The occupational therapist notices on assessment that an area over the patient's left elbow appears as non-blanchable erythema and the skin is intact. The occupational therapist should score the patient as having which of the following?**

    a. Stage I pressure ulcer
    b. Stage II pressure ulcer
    c. Stage III pressure ulcer
    d. Stage IV pressure ulcer

47. A newborn baby exhibits a reflex that includes: hand opening, abducted and extended extremities following a jarring motion. Which of the following correctly identifies the reflex?

    a.  ATNR reflex
    b.  Startle reflex
    c.  Grasping reflex
    d.  Moro reflex

48. An occupational therapist suspects a patient is developing Bell's Palsy. The occupational therapist wants to test the function of cranial nerve VII. Which of the following would be the most appropriate testing procedures?

    a.  Test the taste sensation over the back of the tongue and activation of the facial muscles.
    b.  Test the taste sensation over the front of the tongue and activation of the facial muscles.
    c.  Test the sensation of the facial muscles and sensation of the back of the tongue.
    d.  Test the sensation of the facial muscles and sensation of the front of the tongue.

49. An occupational therapist is reviewing a patient's serum glucose levels. Which of the following scenarios would indicate abnormal serum glucose values for a 30-year-old male?

    a.  70 mg/dl
    b.  55 mg/dl
    c.  110 mg/dl
    d.  100 mg/dl

50. A two-year old has been in the hospital for 3 weeks and seldom seen family members due to isolation precautions. Which of the following hospitalization changes is most like to be occurring?

    a.  Guilt
    b.  Trust
    c.  Separation anxiety
    d.  Shame

51. An occupational therapist is working in a pediatric clinic and a 25-year-old mother comes in with a 12-week-old baby for initial evaluation. The mother is stress out about loss of sleep and the baby exhibits signs of colic. Which of the following techniques should the occupational therapist teach the mother?

    a.  Distraction of the infant with a red object
    b.  Prone positioning techniques
    c.  Tapping reflex techniques
    d.  Neural warmth techniques

52. An occupational therapist is working in a pediatric clinic and a mother brings in her 13-month-old child who has Down Syndrome. The mother reports, "My child's muscles feel weak and he isn't moving well. My RN friend check his reflexes and she said they are diminished." Which of the following actions should the occupational therapist take first?

    a.  Contact the physician immediately
    b.  Have the patient go to X-ray for a c-spine work-up.
    c.  Start an IV on the patient
    d.  Position the child's neck in a neutral position

**53. An occupational therapist is evaluating a child's voluntary release of a toy? Complete release that is voluntary should occur by?**

- a. 6 months
- b. 8 months
- c. 10 months
- d. 12 months

**54. A 29-year-old male has a diagnosis of AIDS. The patient has had a two-year history of AIDS. The most like cognitive deficits include which of the following?**

- a. Disorientation
- b. Sensory changes
- c. Inability to produce sound
- d. Hearing deficits

**55. Which of the following is not a sign or symptom caused by cubital tunnel syndrome?**

- a. Loss of lumbricals
- b. Paresthesia in digit V.
- c. Pain with elbow flexion
- d. Abnormal Flexor carpi ulnaris strength

**56. Which of the following medications is not considered a neuromuscular blocker?**

- a. Anectine
- b. Pavulon
- c. Pitressin
- d. Mivacron

**57. An occupational therapist is caring for a 10-year-old boy who has just been diagnosed with a congenital heart defect. Which of the following clinical signs does not indicate CHF?**

- a. Increased body weight
- b. Elevated heart rate
- c. Lower extremity edema
- d. Compulsive behavior

**58. An occupational therapist working in a pediatric clinic and observes the following situations. Which of the following may indicate a delayed child to the occupational therapist?**

- a. A 12-month old that does not "cruise".
- b. A 8-month old that can sit upright unsupported.
- c. A 6-month old that is rolling prone to supine.
- d. A 3-month old that does not roll supine to prone.

**59. An occupational therapist is reviewing a patient's current Lithium levels. Which of the following values is outside the therapeutic range?**

- a. 1.0 mEq/L
- b. 1.1 mEq/L
- c. 1.2 mEq/L
- d. 1.3 mEq/L

**60. Which of the following describes radial tunnel syndrome?**

    a. Compression of the Anterior Interosseous Nerve
    b. Compression of the Posterior Interosseous Nerve
    c. Crutch Palsy
    d. Cubital Tunnel Syndrome

**61. A patient has been ordered to get Klonopin for the first time. Which of the following side effects is not associated with Klonopin?**

    a. Drowsiness
    b. Ataxia
    c. Salivation elevated
    d. Diplopia

**62. A patient has been diagnosed with diabetes mellitus. Which of the following is not a clinical sign of diabetes mellitus?**

    a. Polyphagia
    b. Polyuria
    c. Metabolic acidosis
    d. Lower extremity edema

**63. A patient has fallen off a bicycle and fractured the distal radius with an avulsion of the ulna styloid. Which of the following terms would apply?**

    a. De Quervain's Syndrome
    b. Colles fracture
    c. Gamekeeper's fracture
    d. Mallet finger

**64. Which of the following motions is identified with the corresponding action?**

**(Action- Turning palm of hand over to face in the anterior direction, dorsum of the hand is pointed downward toward the floor.)**

    a. Pronation
    b. Supination
    c. Abduction
    d. Adduction

**65. An occupational therapist is caring for a retired MD. The MD asks the question, "What type of cells secrete insulin?" The correct answer is:**

    a. alpha cells
    b. beta cells
    c. CD4 cells
    d. helper cells

**66. Which of the following is not considered one of the main mechanisms of Type II Diabetes treatment?**

    a. Medications
    b. Nutrition
    c. Increased activity
    d. Continuous Insulin

**67. An occupational therapist is caring for a retired MD. The MD asks the question, "What type of cells create exocrine secretions?" The correct answer is:**

a. alpha cells
b. beta cells
c. acinar cells
d. plasma cells

**68. An occupational therapist is caring for a patient who has experienced burns to the right upper extremity. According to the Rule of Nines which of the following percentages most accurately describes the severity of the injury?**

a. 36%
b. 27%
c. 18%
d. 9%

**69. A patient has experienced a severe third degree burn to the trunk in the last 36 hours. Which phase of burn management is the patient in?**

a. Shock phase
b. Emergent phase
c. Healing phase
d. Wound proliferation phase

**70. An occupational therapist is reviewing a patient's medical record. The record indicates the patient has limited shoulder flexion on the left. Which plane of movement is limited?**

a. Horizontal
b. Sagittal
c. Frontal
d. Vertical

**71. A client is 72 hours post-op a TKR surgery. The occupational therapist notices that 270 cc's of sero-sanguinous accumulates in the surgical drains. What action should the occupational therapist take?**

a. Notify the doctor
b. Empty the drain
c. Do nothing
d. Remove the drain

**72. An occupational therapist is assigned to do home education teaching to a blind patient who is scheduled for discharge the following morning. What teaching strategy would best fit the situation?**

a. Verbal teaching in short sessions throughout the day
b. Pre-operative booklet on the surgery in Braille
c. Provide a tape for the client
d. Have the blind patient's family member instruct the patient.

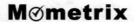

**73. A violation of a patient's confidentiality occurs if two occupational therapists are discussing client information in which of the following scenarios?**

    a.  With an occupational therapist treating the patient

    b.  With a social worker planning for discharge

    c.  With another occupational therapist on duty to plan for break time

    d.  In the hallway outside the patient's room.

**74. If your patient is acutely psychotic, which of the following independent interventions would not be appropriate?**

    a.  Conveying calmness with one on one interaction

    b.  Recognizing and dealing with your own feelings to prevent escalation of the patient's anxiety level

    c.  Encourage client participation in group therapy

    d.  Listen and identify causes of their behavior

**75. An occupational therapist runs into the significant other of a patient with end stage AIDS crying during her smoke break. Which of the following is most appropriate action for the occupational therapist to take?**

    a.  Allow her to grieve by herself.

    b.  Tell her go ahead and cry, after all your husband's pretty bad off.

    c.  Tell her you realize how upset she is, but you don't want to talk about it now.

    d.  Approach her, offering tissues and encourage her to verbalize her feelings.

# Answer Key and Explanations

**1. B:** Teres Minor, Infraspinatus, Supraspinatus, and Subscapularis make up the Rotator Cuff.

**2. B:** The patient experiencing neurovascular changes should have the highest priority. Pain following a TKR is normal, and breakdown over the heels is a gradual process. Moreover, a subacute ankle sprain is almost never a medical emergency.

**3. B:** Gamekeeper's thumb identifies this condition.

**4. B:** Pain may be indicating neurovascular complication.

**5. B:** Stimulation in the form of pictures may decrease signs of confusion.

**6. D:** Adolescents exhibiting signs of sexual development and interest are normal.

**7. A:** Aides should be competent on transfers.

**8. D:** All protective measures must be worn; it is not required to double glove.

**9. A:** Total flexion minus total extension = TAM score.

**10. C:** Both the family and the patient should have the need for restraints explained to them.

**11. B:** The suicide plan may have been decided.

**12. A:** Thrush may be occurring and the patient may need Nystatin.

**13. B:** Check the intake and output prior to making any decisions about patient care.

**14. A:** Negative culture results would indicate absence of infection.

**15. A:** Purse lip breathing will help decrease the volume of air expelled by increased bronchial airways.

**16. B:** The Mantoux is the most accurate test to determine the presence of TB.

**17. D:** The MRI will require supine positioning.

**18. A:** The frontal lobe is responsible for behavior and emotions.

**19. C:** The patient's safety should have the highest priority.

**20. A:** Seclusion is your best option in this scenario.

**21. A:** CBAN, cold, burn, ache, numbness

**22. B:** A ninhydrin test is used to check a patient's ability to sweat.

**23. D:** The patient is in a state of denial.

**24. B:** Fainting and hypotension can be caused by Tricyclics.

**25. B:** Palpitations and muscle weakness are found with excessive levels of Digitalis.

**26. B:** All of the clinical signs indicate a hyperglycemic condition.

**27. D:** Anxiety is a clinical sign associated with respiratory acidosis.

**28. D:** <200 T4 cells/deciliter

**29. C:** Contacting the attending physician via the medical record is appropriate due to the possibility of melanoma.

**30. A:** The patient is at high risk of developing increased intracranial pressure (ICP).

**31. B:** The time slots and daily container would be the best recommendation in this case.

**32. C:** Muscle weakness in the lower extremities is found in acute cases of Guillain-Barre' Syndrome.

**33. A:** The shunt may be blocked and require immediate medical attention.

**34. A:** LOC is the most critical indicator of impaired neurological capabilities.

**35. A:** Patient safety should be the top concern about this patient.

**36. B:** Unilateral pupil changes indicate changes in ICP.

**37. D:** Left sided heart failure exhibits signs of pulmonary compromise (SOB).

**38. C:** Some facilities require the physician to be notified about a patient's request and written permission from the husband is required for the wife to view the chart.

**39. D:** Meal preparation is a multi-level problem solving situation.

**40. A:** Hypotension may be result of over correction of a hypertensive condition.

**41. B:** All of these criteria match up with a Swan Neck Deformity.

**42. C:** Calcium is the most recognized osteoporosis treatment.

**43. D:** Atropine encourages increased rate of conduction in the AV node.

**44. B:** Lidocaine Hydrochloride can cause fatigue and confusion if an over dosage occurs.

**45. D:** The spinner knob is your best recommendation given these parameters.

**46. A:** Erythema with the skin intact can indicate a Stage I pressure ulcer.

**47. D:** The moro reflex has all of the listed characteristics.

**48. B:** The facial nerve (VII) is motor to the face and sensory to the anterior tongue.

**49. B:** 60-115 mg/dl is standard range for serum glucose levels.

**50. C:** Separation anxiety can easily occur after six months during hospitalization.

**51. D:** Neural warmth will help to lower the baby's agitation level.

**52. D:** An atlanto-axial dislocation may have occurred. Position the child in a neutral c-spine posture and then contact the doctor immediately.

**53. D:** At one year this skill should be developed.

**54. A:** Cognitive changes may include confusion and disorientation.

**55. A:** FCU strength is fine in most cases.

**56. C:** Pitressin is a hormone replacement medication.

**57. D:** Compulsive behavior does not indicate CHF.

**58. A:** At 12 months a child should at least be "cruising" (holding on to objects to walk). Cruising is considered pre-walking.

**59. D:** 1.0-1.2 mEq/L is considered standard therapeutic range for patient care.

**60. B:** Posterior Interosseous Nerve compression can cause RTS.

**61. D:** A-C are associated side effects of Klonopin.

**62. D:** A-C are associated with diabetes mellitus.

**63. B:** These descriptions match up with a Colles fracture.

**64. B:** Supination- "Holding a bowl of soup in your hand."

**65. B:** Beta cells secrete insulin.

**66. D:** Insulin is not required in continuous treatment for every Type II diabetic.

**67. C:** Acinar cells create exocrine secretions.

**68. D:** Each arm is scored as 9% according to the Rule of Nines.

**69. A:** The shock phase is considered the first 24-48 hours in wound management.

**70. B:** Sagittal motion occurs in the midline plane of the body.

**71. A:** The physician should be notified if excessive drainage is noted from the surgical site.

**72. A:** Information is smaller amounts is easier to retain. Teaching the day before the discharge is best accomplished in a one on one format.

**73. D:** Hallway discussions should not occur, because you do not who is listening, even though it may be a professional discussion.

**74. C:** Acutely psychotic patients will disrupt group activities.

**75. D:** Being left alone during the grief process, isolates individuals. These individuals need an outlet for their feelings and to talk to someone who is empathetic.

# Image Credits

## LICENSED UNDER CC BY 3.0 (CREATIVECOMMONS.ORG/LICENSES/BY/3.0/)

Planes of the Body: "Planes of the Body" by OpenStax College (https://commons.wikimedia.org/wiki/File:Planes_of_Body.jpg)

Flexion and Extension: "Flexion and Extension" by OpenStax College (https://commons.wikimedia.org/wiki/File:Flexion_and_extension.jpg)

Eversion and Inversion: "Eversion and Inversion" by OpenStax College (https://commons.wikimedia.org/wiki/File:Eversion_and_inversion.jpg)

Pronation and Supination: "Pronation and Supination" by OpenStax College (https://commons.wikimedia.org/wiki/File:Pronation_and_supination.jpg)

Body Movements: "Abduction and Adduction" by OpenStax College (https://commons.wikimedia.org/wiki/File:Body_Movements_I.jpg)

## LICENSED UNDER CC BY-SA 3.0 (CREATIVECOMMONS.ORG/LICENSES/BY-SA/3.0/)

Body Movements: "Abduction and Adduction" by OpenStax College (https://commons.wikimedia.org/wiki/File:Body_Movements_I_(cropped_AbAd).jpg)

## PUBLIC DOMAIN

Lund-Browder Chart-Burn Injury Area: "Rule of Nines" by U.S. Department of Health and Human Services (https://commons.wikimedia.org/wiki/File:Lund-Browder_chart-burn_injury_area.PNG)

## CREDITED

Grips: "Types of Prehension" by Digital Resource Foundation for the Orthotics & Prosthetics Community (http://www.oandplibrary.org/al/1955_02_022.asp)

# How to Overcome Test Anxiety

Just the thought of taking a test is enough to make most people a little nervous. A test is an important event that can have a long-term impact on your future, so it's important to take it seriously and it's natural to feel anxious about performing well. But just because anxiety is normal, that doesn't mean that it's helpful in test taking, or that you should simply accept it as part of your life. Anxiety can have a variety of effects. These effects can be mild, like making you feel slightly nervous, or severe, like blocking your ability to focus or remember even a simple detail.

If you experience test anxiety—whether severe or mild—it's important to know how to beat it. To discover this, first you need to understand what causes test anxiety.

## Causes of Test Anxiety

While we often think of anxiety as an uncontrollable emotional state, it can actually be caused by simple, practical things. One of the most common causes of test anxiety is that a person does not feel adequately prepared for their test. This feeling can be the result of many different issues such as poor study habits or lack of organization, but the most common culprit is time management. Starting to study too late, failing to organize your study time to cover all of the material, or being distracted while you study will mean that you're not well prepared for the test. This may lead to cramming the night before, which will cause you to be physically and mentally exhausted for the test. Poor time management also contributes to feelings of stress, fear, and hopelessness as you realize you are not well prepared but don't know what to do about it.

Other times, test anxiety is not related to your preparation for the test but comes from unresolved fear. This may be a past failure on a test, or poor performance on tests in general. It may come from comparing yourself to others who seem to be performing better or from the stress of living up to expectations. Anxiety may be driven by fears of the future—how failure on this test would affect your educational and career goals. These fears are often completely irrational, but they can still negatively impact your test performance.

> **Review Video: <u>3 Reasons You Have Test Anxiety</u>**
> Visit mometrix.com/academy and enter code: 428468

# Elements of Test Anxiety

As mentioned earlier, test anxiety is considered to be an emotional state, but it has physical and mental components as well. Sometimes you may not even realize that you are suffering from test anxiety until you notice the physical symptoms. These can include trembling hands, rapid heartbeat, sweating, nausea, and tense muscles. Extreme anxiety may lead to fainting or vomiting. Obviously, any of these symptoms can have a negative impact on testing. It is important to recognize them as soon as they begin to occur so that you can address the problem before it damages your performance.

> **Review Video: 3 Ways to Tell You Have Test Anxiety**
> Visit mometrix.com/academy and enter code: 927847

The mental components of test anxiety include trouble focusing and inability to remember learned information. During a test, your mind is on high alert, which can help you recall information and stay focused for an extended period of time. However, anxiety interferes with your mind's natural processes, causing you to blank out, even on the questions you know well. The strain of testing during anxiety makes it difficult to stay focused, especially on a test that may take several hours. Extreme anxiety can take a huge mental toll, making it difficult not only to recall test information but even to understand the test questions or pull your thoughts together.

> **Review Video: How Test Anxiety Affects Memory**
> Visit mometrix.com/academy and enter code: 609003

# Effects of Test Anxiety

Test anxiety is like a disease—if left untreated, it will get progressively worse. Anxiety leads to poor performance, and this reinforces the feelings of fear and failure, which in turn lead to poor performances on subsequent tests. It can grow from a mild nervousness to a crippling condition. If allowed to progress, test anxiety can have a big impact on your schooling, and consequently on your future.

Test anxiety can spread to other parts of your life. Anxiety on tests can become anxiety in any stressful situation, and blanking on a test can turn into panicking in a job situation. But fortunately, you don't have to let anxiety rule your testing and determine your grades. There are a number of relatively simple steps you can take to move past anxiety and function normally on a test and in the rest of life.

> **Review Video: How Test Anxiety Impacts Your Grades**
> Visit mometrix.com/academy and enter code: 939819

# Physical Steps for Beating Test Anxiety

While test anxiety is a serious problem, the good news is that it can be overcome. It doesn't have to control your ability to think and remember information. While it may take time, you can begin taking steps today to beat anxiety.

Just as your first hint that you may be struggling with anxiety comes from the physical symptoms, the first step to treating it is also physical. Rest is crucial for having a clear, strong mind. If you are tired, it is much easier to give in to anxiety. But if you establish good sleep habits, your body and mind will be ready to perform optimally, without the strain of exhaustion. Additionally, sleeping well helps you to retain information better, so you're more likely to recall the answers when you see the test questions.

Getting good sleep means more than going to bed on time. It's important to allow your brain time to relax. Take study breaks from time to time so it doesn't get overworked, and don't study right before bed. Take time to rest your mind before trying to rest your body, or you may find it difficult to fall asleep.

> **Review Video: <u>The Importance of Sleep for Your Brain</u>**
> Visit mometrix.com/academy and enter code: 319338

Along with sleep, other aspects of physical health are important in preparing for a test. Good nutrition is vital for good brain function. Sugary foods and drinks may give a burst of energy but this burst is followed by a crash, both physically and emotionally. Instead, fuel your body with protein and vitamin-rich foods.

Also, drink plenty of water. Dehydration can lead to headaches and exhaustion, especially if your brain is already under stress from the rigors of the test. Particularly if your test is a long one, drink water during the breaks. And if possible, take an energy-boosting snack to eat between sections.

> **Review Video: <u>How Diet Can Affect your Mood</u>**
> Visit mometrix.com/academy and enter code: 624317

Along with sleep and diet, a third important part of physical health is exercise. Maintaining a steady workout schedule is helpful, but even taking 5-minute study breaks to walk can help get your blood pumping faster and clear your head. Exercise also releases endorphins, which contribute to a positive feeling and can help combat test anxiety.

When you nurture your physical health, you are also contributing to your mental health. If your body is healthy, your mind is much more likely to be healthy as well. So take time to rest, nourish your body with healthy food and water, and get moving as much as possible. Taking these physical steps will make you stronger and more able to take the mental steps necessary to overcome test anxiety.

# Mental Steps for Beating Test Anxiety

Working on the mental side of test anxiety can be more challenging, but as with the physical side, there are clear steps you can take to overcome it. As mentioned earlier, test anxiety often stems from lack of preparation, so the obvious solution is to prepare for the test. Effective studying may be the most important weapon you have for beating test anxiety, but you can and should employ several other mental tools to combat fear.

First, boost your confidence by reminding yourself of past success—tests or projects that you aced. If you're putting as much effort into preparing for this test as you did for those, there's no reason you should expect to fail here. Work hard to prepare; then trust your preparation.

Second, surround yourself with encouraging people. It can be helpful to find a study group, but be sure that the people you're around will encourage a positive attitude. If you spend time with others who are anxious or cynical, this will only contribute to your own anxiety. Look for others who are motivated to study hard from a desire to succeed, not from a fear of failure.

Third, reward yourself. A test is physically and mentally tiring, even without anxiety, and it can be helpful to have something to look forward to. Plan an activity following the test, regardless of the outcome, such as going to a movie or getting ice cream.

When you are taking the test, if you find yourself beginning to feel anxious, remind yourself that you know the material. Visualize successfully completing the test. Then take a few deep, relaxing breaths and return to it. Work through the questions carefully but with confidence, knowing that you are capable of succeeding.

Developing a healthy mental approach to test taking will also aid in other areas of life. Test anxiety affects more than just the actual test—it can be damaging to your mental health and even contribute to depression. It's important to beat test anxiety before it becomes a problem for more than testing.

---

**Review Video: <u>Test Anxiety and Depression</u>**
Visit mometrix.com/academy and enter code: 904704

---

# Study Strategy

Being prepared for the test is necessary to combat anxiety, but what does being prepared look like? You may study for hours on end and still not feel prepared. What you need is a strategy for test prep. The next few pages outline our recommended steps to help you plan out and conquer the challenge of preparation.

## STEP 1: SCOPE OUT THE TEST

Learn everything you can about the format (multiple choice, essay, etc.) and what will be on the test. Gather any study materials, course outlines, or sample exams that may be available. Not only will this help you to prepare, but knowing what to expect can help to alleviate test anxiety.

## STEP 2: MAP OUT THE MATERIAL

Look through the textbook or study guide and make note of how many chapters or sections it has. Then divide these over the time you have. For example, if a book has 15 chapters and you have five days to study, you need to cover three chapters each day. Even better, if you have the time, leave an extra day at the end for overall review after you have gone through the material in depth.

If time is limited, you may need to prioritize the material. Look through it and make note of which sections you think you already have a good grasp on, and which need review. While you are studying, skim quickly through the familiar sections and take more time on the challenging parts. Write out your plan so you don't get lost as you go. Having a written plan also helps you feel more in control of the study, so anxiety is less likely to arise from feeling overwhelmed at the amount to cover.

## STEP 3: GATHER YOUR TOOLS

Decide what study method works best for you. Do you prefer to highlight in the book as you study and then go back over the highlighted portions? Or do you type out notes of the important information? Or is it helpful to make flashcards that you can carry with you? Assemble the pens, index cards, highlighters, post-it notes, and any other materials you may need so you won't be distracted by getting up to find things while you study.

If you're having a hard time retaining the information or organizing your notes, experiment with different methods. For example, try color-coding by subject with colored pens, highlighters, or post-it notes. If you learn better by hearing, try recording yourself reading your notes so you can listen while in the car, working out, or simply sitting at your desk. Ask a friend to quiz you from your flashcards, or try teaching someone the material to solidify it in your mind.

## STEP 4: CREATE YOUR ENVIRONMENT

It's important to avoid distractions while you study. This includes both the obvious distractions like visitors and the subtle distractions like an uncomfortable chair (or a too-comfortable couch that makes you want to fall asleep). Set up the best study environment possible: good lighting and a comfortable work area. If background music helps you focus, you may want to turn it on, but otherwise keep the room quiet. If you are using a computer to take notes, be sure you don't have any other windows open, especially applications like social media, games, or anything else that could distract you. Silence your phone and turn off notifications. Be sure to keep water close by so you stay hydrated while you study (but avoid unhealthy drinks and snacks).

Also, take into account the best time of day to study. Are you freshest first thing in the morning? Try to set aside some time then to work through the material. Is your mind clearer in the afternoon or evening? Schedule your study session then. Another method is to study at the same time of day that you will take the test, so that your brain gets used to working on the material at that time and will be ready to focus at test time.

## STEP 5: STUDY!

Once you have done all the study preparation, it's time to settle into the actual studying. Sit down, take a few moments to settle your mind so you can focus, and begin to follow your study plan. Don't give in to distractions or let yourself procrastinate. This is your time to prepare so you'll be ready to fearlessly approach the test. Make the most of the time and stay focused.

Of course, you don't want to burn out. If you study too long you may find that you're not retaining the information very well. Take regular study breaks. For example, taking five minutes out of every hour to walk briskly, breathing deeply and swinging your arms, can help your mind stay fresh.

As you get to the end of each chapter or section, it's a good idea to do a quick review. Remind yourself of what you learned and work on any difficult parts. When you feel that you've mastered the material, move on to the next part. At the end of your study session, briefly skim through your notes again.

But while review is helpful, cramming last minute is NOT. If at all possible, work ahead so that you won't need to fit all your study into the last day. Cramming overloads your brain with more information than it can process and retain, and your tired mind may struggle to recall even previously learned information when it is overwhelmed with last-minute study. Also, the urgent nature of cramming and the stress placed on your brain contribute to anxiety. You'll be more likely to go to the test feeling unprepared and having trouble thinking clearly.

So don't cram, and don't stay up late before the test, even just to review your notes at a leisurely pace. Your brain needs rest more than it needs to go over the information again. In fact, plan to finish your studies by noon or early afternoon the day before the test. Give your brain the rest of the day to relax or focus on other things, and get a good night's sleep. Then you will be fresh for the test and better able to recall what you've studied.

## STEP 6: TAKE A PRACTICE TEST

Many courses offer sample tests, either online or in the study materials. This is an excellent resource to check whether you have mastered the material, as well as to prepare for the test format and environment.

Check the test format ahead of time: the number of questions, the type (multiple choice, free response, etc.), and the time limit. Then create a plan for working through them. For example, if you have 30 minutes to take a 60-question test, your limit is 30 seconds per question. Spend less time on the questions you know well so that you can take more time on the difficult ones.

If you have time to take several practice tests, take the first one open book, with no time limit. Work through the questions at your own pace and make sure you fully understand them. Gradually work up to taking a test under test conditions: sit at a desk with all study materials put away and set a timer. Pace yourself to make sure you finish the test with time to spare and go back to check your answers if you have time.

After each test, check your answers. On the questions you missed, be sure you understand why you missed them. Did you misread the question (tests can use tricky wording)? Did you forget the information? Or was it something you hadn't learned? Go back and study any shaky areas that the practice tests reveal.

Taking these tests not only helps with your grade, but also aids in combating test anxiety. If you're already used to the test conditions, you're less likely to worry about it, and working through tests until you're scoring well gives you a confidence boost. Go through the practice tests until you feel comfortable, and then you can go into the test knowing that you're ready for it.

## Test Tips

On test day, you should be confident, knowing that you've prepared well and are ready to answer the questions. But aside from preparation, there are several test day strategies you can employ to maximize your performance.

First, as stated before, get a good night's sleep the night before the test (and for several nights before that, if possible). Go into the test with a fresh, alert mind rather than staying up late to study.

Try not to change too much about your normal routine on the day of the test. It's important to eat a nutritious breakfast, but if you normally don't eat breakfast at all, consider eating just a protein bar. If you're a coffee drinker, go ahead and have your normal coffee. Just make sure you time it so that the caffeine doesn't wear off right in the middle of your test. Avoid sugary beverages, and drink enough water to stay hydrated but not so much that you need a restroom break 10 minutes into the test. If your test isn't first thing in the morning, consider going for a walk or doing a light workout before the test to get your blood flowing.

Allow yourself enough time to get ready, and leave for the test with plenty of time to spare so you won't have the anxiety of scrambling to arrive in time. Another reason to be early is to select a good seat. It's helpful to sit away from doors and windows, which can be distracting. Find a good seat, get out your supplies, and settle your mind before the test begins.

When the test begins, start by going over the instructions carefully, even if you already know what to expect. Make sure you avoid any careless mistakes by following the directions.

Then begin working through the questions, pacing yourself as you've practiced. If you're not sure on an answer, don't spend too much time on it, and don't let it shake your confidence. Either skip it and come back later, or eliminate as many wrong answers as possible and guess among the remaining ones. Don't dwell on these questions as you continue—put them out of your mind and focus on what lies ahead.

Be sure to read all of the answer choices, even if you're sure the first one is the right answer. Sometimes you'll find a better one if you keep reading. But don't second-guess yourself if you do immediately know the answer. Your gut instinct is usually right. Don't let test anxiety rob you of the information you know.

If you have time at the end of the test (and if the test format allows), go back and review your answers. Be cautious about changing any, since your first instinct tends to be correct, but make sure you didn't misread any of the questions or accidentally mark the wrong answer choice. Look over any you skipped and make an educated guess.

At the end, leave the test feeling confident. You've done your best, so don't waste time worrying about your performance or wishing you could change anything. Instead, celebrate the successful

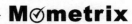

completion of this test. And finally, use this test to learn how to deal with anxiety even better next time.

> **Review Video: 5 Tips to Beat Test Anxiety**
> Visit mometrix.com/academy and enter code: 570656

## Important Qualification

Not all anxiety is created equal. If your test anxiety is causing major issues in your life beyond the classroom or testing center, or if you are experiencing troubling physical symptoms related to your anxiety, it may be a sign of a serious physiological or psychological condition. If this sounds like your situation, we strongly encourage you to seek professional help.

# Thank You

We at Mometrix would like to extend our heartfelt thanks to you, our friend and patron, for allowing us to play a part in your journey. It is a privilege to serve people from all walks of life who are unified in their commitment to building the best future they can for themselves.

The preparation you devote to these important testing milestones may be the most valuable educational opportunity you have for making a real difference in your life. We encourage you to put your heart into it—that feeling of succeeding, overcoming, and yes, conquering will be well worth the hours you've invested.

We want to hear your story, your struggles and your successes, and if you see any opportunities for us to improve our materials so we can help others even more effectively in the future, please share that with us as well. **The team at Mometrix would be absolutely thrilled to hear from you!** So please, send us an email (support@mometrix.com) and let's stay in touch.

> **If you'd like some additional help, check out these other resources we offer for your exam:**
> http://mometrixflashcards.com/NBCOT

163

# Additional Bonus Material

Due to our efforts to try to keep this book to a manageable length, we've created a link that will give you access to all of your additional bonus material:

**mometrix.com/bonus948/ot**